CW00967911

Healing

With

Sondra Ray

Medicine Bear Publishing
Blue Hill, Maine

Medicine Bear Publishing
P.O. Box 1075
Blue Hill, ME 04614

Cover Art by Isabelle Rudolphi

Printed in the United States

ISBN 0-9651546-6-1

Library of Congress CCN 97-070855

First Printing 1997
Printed in the United States

I dedicate this book to my Mother,
Ethel Miller...
who has allowed me to be different,
who taught me very high thoughts,
and always grounded me in strength.

Contents

PART I

Background

Dedication to my Colleagues

This book is dedicated to all my colleagues in the Healing Arts who have given me so much support for the last two decades. I thank them for their expertise, commitment and service to humanity - and all their personal help to me!

I also thank all healers who are dedicated to their work and I hope to meet them and experience their work. It is through our sharing that we create ever-larger networks of unity.

I am including this dedication as a part of the "Background" section of this book because each one of these outstanding healers has contributed in large measure to my learning-healing background.

Spiritual Guides and Healers:
Gerardo Pizzaro (Spain)
Jose Luis Perez (Spain)
Elena Duranona (Spain)
Barbara Wilson (Australia)
Jenny Putman (Australia)
Carol Elliot (Australia)
Doris Ankarberg (Sweden)
Virginia Fidel (Montana)
Genni Wallace (Washington State)
Kerry Henwood (California)
Jeannie Loomis (Connecticut)
Ruth Green (Philadelphia)
Janolyn (California)
Susan Drew (California)
Beatrix Quintana (Sedona, Arizona)
Ivelisse Cintron (Puerto Rico)
Gabriella De Lange (Atlanta, Georgia)
Marti Klabunde (Iowa)

Beth Hin (Santa Fe, New Mexico)
Leslie Thurston (Santa Fe, New Mexico)
Rama Vernon (Sedona)

Kahunas:
Mornnah Simeona (Hawaii...passed over)
Al Kahekeliula (Hawaii)
Sherman Dudoit (Maui, Hawaii)

Body Workers:
Don McFarland: Founder of Body Harmony (California)
Patrick Collard: Body Magic (California)
Arne Rantzen (Boston)
Joe Heller: Heller Work (California)

Rolfing:
Veronique: My Original Rolfer (California)
Kermit Stick (Nova Scotia)
Howard Finklestein (New York)
Giselle Genillard (Santa Fe)

Chiropractors:
Reza Samvat (Australia)
Alan Lazar (California)
Michael McBride (Hawaii)
Joe Adler (New York City)
Dr. Pick (Los Angeles)
Dr. Dominique (London)
Dr. Ernest Loveland (Puerto Rico)
* See special tribute to Network Chiopractors in final chapter.

Osteopathy:
Dr. Upledger (Florida)
Dr. Anthony Bryant (New Zealand)
Marino Martin (Madrid, Spain)
Walt Wirth (Indianapolis)

Acupuncture:
Dr. Daniel Mene (Paris, France)
Dr. Michael Oddon (Aux en Provence, France)
Dr. Chen (Los Angeles)
Dr. SLK Cheung (London)
Dr. Martin Orimenko (St. Louis, Mo.)
Vicky Woolger (Gold Coast, Australia)
Vivian Lee (Palm Desert, Ca.)
Dairne McLoughlin (Albuquerque, NM)

Reflexology and Nutrition:
Michealangelo Chiechi (Milan, Italy)

Energy Medicine:
Dr. Linda Lancaster (Santa Fe)

Medical Doctors:
Dr. Bob Doughton (Portland)
Dr. Roy Jones (Denver)
Dr. Bruce Roseman (New York City)
Dr. Sandip Mukerjee (New Delhi, India)

Therapist-Hypnotist:
Dr. Irv Katz (Maui, Hawaii)

Dentist:
Dr. Neil McLeod (Los Angeles)

Rebirthers:
A special thanks to Leonard Orr, Founder of Rebirthing
 (See back of book for contacting Rebirthers in your area)

LRT Trainers
Bob Mandel (former director and partner for LRT)
Mallie Mandel
Michael Fatjo (first LRT trainer after myself)
Fredric Lehrman
Diane Hinterman

Paul and Layne Cutright
Peter and Meg Kane
Vince and Yve Betar
Philip and Mikela Tarlow
Bob and Mallie Mandel
Claudia Kaplan
Arne Rantzen

Current LRT Trainers:
Rhonda Le Vand Baker
Lea Adler
Diane Roberts
Patrice Ellequain
Kelly Walden
Bernd Shroeder
Sondra Ray
Debbie Miller
Thanks to all the LRT Trainers and to all who worked so hard to produce and organize the LRT training events!

My Personal Gurus:
Jesus
Babaji
Amaji
Shastriji
Muniraj
Mother Mary
Mother Meera
My Mother, Ethel Miller
The Divine Mother

I honor ADOLFO DOMINIGUES, producer and Rebirther in Madrid, Spain, who opened his home to me while I was writing this book and who has been responsible for my loving and constant support system in Spain. He has brought into my life some of the greatest healers I have ever known.

A special thanks to the women who took care of me privately during initiations:

Emily Goldman (Santa Fe)
Shanti (France)
Terry Battle (Puerto Rico)
Janine D'Andrade (California)
Kate Garrity (Puerto Rico)
Special mention to my personal Rebirther, Coordinator and Friend
Sharda Collard.

*And a special tribute to Network Chiopractic
 (see P. 232-235)

I thank my publisher Jonathon Ray.

Foreword

My master, Babaji, always used to say to those of us who had come to India, "I could heal you all instantly, but what would you learn?"

So then, we would have to learn to work out our problems by ourselves. Of course, we always learned much more quickly with Babaji's support. And often he would take pity on us and take on some of our karma in order to lighten our load. With and without Babaji's guidance, I certainly have had my share of "learning experiences" that I do not care to repeat. Somehow I have been good at helping others to heal themselves, but I have not been such a good healer for myself. In fact, even though I have been a healer since day one, I was hesitant to write a book on this subject until I felt myself reasonably well-healed.

Even though there was a miracle at my birth - my grandfather was instantly healed at the sight of me - I always felt that I had failed because of my father's death. My father was sick during most of my life and I took care of him often, starting when I was only three years old. When I was six, I told him exactly how to heal himself! That was to much of a shock for my family and I was reprimanded for being so presumptuous. Watching him slowly dying day-by-day was devastating.

My preoccupation with healing started with my childhood conditioning. I became a nurse in order to understand why people get sick and die, but I did not find the answers that I was intuitively looking for in Western medicine. I wanted to see Permanent Healing, not the same symptoms recurring in patients who were returning to hospitals again and again. I desperately wanted to know how to prevent disease and death.

I was taught that the Bible said, "In God, all things are possible." I took this promise literally and believed that therefore, as a child of God, I deserved to know how to be permanently healed and how to live forever! If all things were possible, surely this included Physical Immortality. After all, there were Immortals mentioned in the Bible.

My father was in and out of hospitals all of my childhood. I have written about this before. What disturbed me most about his chronic illness was that "modern" medicine and religion failed him. He died - and I did not understand why. Later, "modern" medicine and religion failed for me as well. And they failed my sister who died of melanoma. I ended up divorced, with my hair falling out and in continual bodily pain which lasted twelve to fourteen years. Nobody in "modern" medicine could help me, so I began searching for other answers.

Finally I was able to begin a real journey of self-healing with alternative methods. But I have had to learn a lot and, basically, re-condition myself about what "healing" really means. This book is an attempt to share with others what I have learned thus far in my healing journey, but it is definitely not my last word on this subject. I am still healing!

I used to blame "modern" medicine and religion. But now I know that "TRUTH CANNOT DEAL WITH ERRORS THAT WE WANT". That statement from the

Course in Miracles is deep enough for a whole chapter alone. Why we want to keep our errors rather than to be healed is a very deep subject. We may think that we want to be healed, but our unconscious sabotage patterns are stronger than we realize. Our challenge is to understand how the unconscious mind works and to learn how to change it. I have written this book for those who really want to be permanently healed and for those who want to help others discover how to do the same.

I wondered, after fourteen books, "How could any book block me as much as this one? How could any book that I would write cause so much commotion? How could any book take so long? What *was* it about this book?" It seemed to have a power of its own - it kept disappearing.

Perhaps it was because I had to face myself even more than when I was writing my other books. Perhaps it was because I had to review parts of my life that I could hardly remember. Perhaps it was because I did not feel healed enough myself to complete it, even though I had healed myself of so many ailments. There always seemed to be more problems coming up and I wanted to be in integrity with what I was writing and really live my words. I guess I was feeling that I was not healed and that I was not whole until every single thing in my life worked perfectly. Maybe I could finally get my body healed, but what about the rest? Maybe my relationships with men were finally working, but what about the money case? (It was atrocious!) I could not get it together. I did not feel healed in my business either. Then, one day I realized that if I waited until everything in my life was working perfectly, I would never get this book out. Maybe Leonard Orr was right when he said that it takes hundreds of years to get your case cracked.

So, on a Palm Sunday in Spain, I began this book again. It is the only book of fourteen that I had to completely re-write twice! Well, I had started it in Spain about four years earlier in the winter. I remember it was cold and I was fed up being without central heating in Old Madrid. Also, it was soon after my sister had died and I was very sad. She had not been healed by her religion and was not interested in alternative techniques. What right did I have to think that I could be permanently healed? It brought back all the memories and emotions of my father's long illness and death. The thought of all that death was overwhelming.

The manuscript got lost. My publishers lost their copy, too. We had a falling out over that. Later I found out that they were very sad, for they had lost an endeared editor to AIDS - the one who used to edit my books! We were all sad and none of us could handle a book on *Permanent Healing* when people we loved were dying.

And yet, that was precisely why I wanted to write this book. Wasn't there any hope? I was holding Jesus to the promise in the Bible: "All things are possible". My higher self was absolutely convinced that it was possible to live in the body free of sickness and pain. I was convinced that we could even stop the aging process if, in fact, "all things were possible". But my lower self had obviously not cleared all the doubts that were in the way of my faith because I still could not get this book back. In time though, it came back. I don't even remember now how we found it because I had lost even the computer discs. Well, I remembered then that this had happened to me once before: Ideal Birth had disappeared twice. When things are not right, they will not happen or they are just gone. They come back when I am ready. My Gurus protect me this way. I had tried to write this book again in Japan at one point in my travels and was really proud that I had started over. I wrote for three days solid on everything I knew about healing. It seemed very comprehensive and I liked my writing style. But, one day - blip!.. it all disappeared again! The book was gone in the computer just like that! A blip like that had always been my worst fear about computers. The hard-drive had failed and I did not have the disc in. I could not understand what was happening. Maybe I had to go through my worst fears and live them out.

Trying to find a computer expert in Japan who spoke English was not easy. The girls that I lived with eventually found someone and he checked my computer forwards and backwards. He phoned me the next day and could only say that he was sorry. The second manuscript, the second attempt at this book, was gone! I admit that I broke down and cried. I had to go through a Rebirthing right then and there.

Thankfully, two of my staff, Veronica and Debbi, were there to Rebirth me. I had to process out more loss. There had been so much loss in my life: everyone dying in my home town, all the funerals that I had to witness, the loss of my father, my sister and the loss of my husband. Could I ever be healed of loss?

So, on that Palm Sunday in Spain, I started this book

for the third time. I really felt that I could push through it. It was spring in Spain and a man I cared for was coming to spend Easter with me. I was also with Adolfo and he was a real balance to my energy. And he was with a beautiful woman, a flamenco dancer whom I really liked. If I was born to be a writer, I had better get on with it no matter what.

In reading my dedication, you might be surprised at the long list of healers that I named. I have, more or less, tried to experience everything possible in the way of alternative healing. My life has been a great transition away from the addiction to Western medicine. It has also been a great learning period. Every one of these people, with various healing techniques, has taught me something new about healing. I have always had a special affinity for healers. I love them as my dearest colleagues for they are quietly working hard in all parts of the world. I have been so blessed to find and meet them, to experience their healing energies and to just hang out with them. Many of them go unacknowledged for their important spiritual service to humanity, and I have tried to acknowledge all of them in this book. I hope that I have not left anyone out. If I have, I hope that I am contacted. My dream, of course, is to somehow get us all together.

Healing Myself

I could have healed myself more quickly had I known, at the times of my "illnesses", all the information that is in this book...especially about the prayer techniques that I have recently discovered. You could say that I traveled the "low road" of trial, error and struggle. This chapter is about that "low road" when I was still addicted to the Western medical models. Remember, I became a nurse and was brainwashed by the conventional system. I was afraid to let go of that system. I thought that I needed doctors in order to survive and it was that dependence that kept me in weakness and helplessness. As you will see, even after I began to give up those Western methods of healing and to explore alternative methods, I was still addicted to struggle. I was making my healing process more difficult than necessary, and I wasted a lot of time worrying that I would never get over some of those symptoms. My constant worry slowed down the healing process considerably.

When I finally became disenchanted with my own profession of medicine, I left it to study spiritual healing. However, even after I left, I was not really "free". I was just rebelling. I became arrogant and canceled all my medical insurance. I went without insurance for ten full years to prove that I would never need a doctor again. But my attitude was not right and, eventually, my arrogance caught up with me. I had a very humbling experience that forced me to go back and forgive Western "modern" medicine for not healing my father.

It took me over a decade to wean myself from the system. I practiced spiritual self-healing as much as possible, but I still sought out medical doctors on a couple of occasions. Realizing that it was going to be a long process to master self-healing totally, I tried to be patient with myself.

Although this book is about how to heal spiritually without the addiction to "modern" medicine, there may be times when one's fear of giving up traditional methods is too great to overcome. In those cases, you might need to go to a doctor. But remember not to limit yourself to traditional methods alone. Try other techniques of healing. Before running to a doctor, you may want to try some of the techniques talked about in this book. The goal, then, is self-healing. Ultimately, the prevention of the disease is the real goal.

I would like to honor all those doctors who have taken my workshops and classes in search of alternative, spiritual healing....Bless You!

What follows is a record of my physical illnesses and what I have learned from those experiences. I am not proud of all the illnesses and negative physical conditions that I have manifested over the years and I wish that learning had been easier. Perhaps the sharing of my healing journey will help others come through their own physical and spiritual healing much faster. But first, let me tell you about my cats!

The Cat Ashram

As a child, I was very lucky for I always got healed by my cats. Believe it or not, I had forty cats at one time! (Of course, my dad would never let them in the house. There were just too many of them.) I guess that I was too busy taking care of all my cats to get very sick.

The temptation to get sick was always very strong in our house, though, as well as in our small Iowa town (population of 300). It seemed that people were dying right and left. The worst part of it all was that all of us children were required to march to the cemetery every time someone died. I took all those deaths very seriously because everyone in my town was my "family" in one sense or another.

Then too, there was my father whom I absolutely adored. He was sick most of the time, and in and out of hospitals. I loved my father and wanted to be just like him, but I did not want to be sick. So, it was a very tricky relationship for me.

When I was twelve, my dad apparently had rheumatic fever. Later, he died of rheumatic heart disease. When he was in the hospital of neighboring Mason City, Iowa, the nuns would never let me in to see him because I was not "old enough". He was always there for a long time, so I used to sneak up the fire escape, crawl through the window and sit with him on the hospital bed. We would usually have just a few minutes together before the nuns would discover me and throw me out.

My dad used to say to the nuns, "You leave her alone". But they never listened and threw me out just the same. He always got better when he saw me. Why is it that the medical profession doesn't realize that children can be healers for their parents?

Again, when I was twelve, I developed all the same symptoms of rheumatic fever that my father had. I got very sick. The doctors could not find any spirochetes nor anything else abnormal in my blood. They told my mother that I had a "pseudo case" - my illness just wasn't real.

"Wow!", I said, "Let me out of here so I can take care of my cats!" I think that experience was the beginning of my body taking on a *lot* of illnesses to make me learn about healing.

My cats always waited for me on my grandparents' porch. I spent a lot of time at their house next door because there was a lot less illness in their home. Whenever my dad would be visiting over there with me , my cats would not budge until I came out and he would have to kick his way through them. As soon as I would come out, they would follow me everywhere except when I rode my bike to town.

We had huge yards, many barns and chicken houses. That was great for the cats and all their litters. Different mother cats had different litters here and there and, somehow, I was in charge of them all - at least I thought so. My cats kept me going. If I felt bad, I could talk to my cats. They would sit on the lawn and patiently listen to me while I gave them long lectures and shared all of my feelings. They would make me feel better and actually heal me. (It was perfect practice for being a public speaker later on. They never interrupted me, walked out or looked bored!) I always felt better after these sessions, and as a child, I was rarely sick except for that one false alarm. I simply did not have time to think about getting sick.

At night when my dad and grandpa used to walk out to the pasture to milk the cows, they would deliberately clang the milk pails together and all the cats would come running. It was like a big parade! My dad and grandpa had a game that they played with my cats. They would aim the cow's teat, full of milk, at a certain cat's mouth. (I always wondered which one would be "chosen".) The cats liked this game and went along with it wholeheartedly and I learned to milk the cows the same way.

Every hay season my grandpa would come over to our house, open the door and yell, "Sondie, there is a new litter of kittens in the hay barn". Then he would shut the door and head for the hayloft. I would run after him as fast as I could and climb up the wooden slats to the loft. There were always so many hay bales piled up in so many ways that it always took me a long time to find the new litter. It was exciting beyond belief, especially when I finally found them.

Sometimes I did not feel that certain mothers were very good cat-mothers and in such cases, when they ignored their young, I had wet-nurses on the side. Blackie was the best surrogate mother and she was always willing to nurse kittens that I felt were ignored. When my Blackie died, old and blind, I was devastated. I held a major funeral for her and all the cats had to attend. After all, that was the way that it was done in our town!

I remember a picture of myself taken on one of my birthdays. My mom had put my angel cake on the sidewalk and the cats came and licked off the frosting. I had long curls with green bows on the tops and the picture reminds me of how I shared everything with my cats. One day my grandpa gave me a big tent and my dad built a wooden floor for it and put in electricity. I had a big bed in there and I was in heaven because then I could sleep with my cats! I was out there even during heavy rain storms. Blackie always got top priority and got to sleep by my face. She was, after all, the best mother and "healer" of my cat family.

My cats were my gurus and my healers when I was young. They took care of me and I took care of them. Even after I went off to college, my cats waited for me to come home. The most amazing thing happened to me when I got older and became a successful writer. My publishers produced a book called *Why Cats Paint*. Phil, the owner of the publishing company, had so much fun doing that book - almost as much fun as I had had as a kid with my cats. He even had a display in the gallery below the publishing house of real, live cats doing paintings while people watched. Apparently, certain cats really do love to paint. (Maybe some of my cats followed me in spirit to the publishing company to write their own books!)

When I left for college and left my cat ashram, all the trouble with my "physical conditions" began. For one thing, my father had just died. He died the night before I was to graduate with honors from high school. I was salutatorian and missed being valedictorian by one point. The salutatorian was required to give the traditional "Message to the Parents". Everyone in town was in the audience, all 300 of them. They all knew my father had just died. I was trying to give a tribute to my dad. I was devastated and frozen in grief. Everyone was crying. My graduation turned into another funeral!

So began a long string of negative physical conditions, and I was forced to deal with issues of health and healing on a very dramatic level. I don't know why I had created so many illnesses in my body during the following years. Maybe it was because I had always been around sick people as a child and I had been unconsciously programmed to repeat the pattern. I used to ride my bike to visit the sick and the elderly in our town. Perhaps even then I was trying to manifest the same illnesses in order to learn about disease. Maybe it was because I had a lot of past-life karma or something, and my death urge got activated. Maybe it was because I was full of anger towards God about death and dying issues. Maybe my strong ego needed to be tamed. Maybe it was my mission in life to become a healer and to master the art of self-healing.

In my adult life, I have created the following illnesses: insomnia, fourteen years of migrating pains, severe hair loss, severe food neurosis, acute arthritis, severe sinusitis, acute hypothermia, melanoma, severe gastritis, rheumatism, paralysis over my heart chakra, several near-death experiences and a few other various and sundry ailments. I have healed these conditions mostly with my mind and alternative methods, except on two occasions when I was so afraid that I lost my faith in spiritual healing. On those two occasions, I turned to "modern medicine", but I eventually realized that my fear had a great power over my physical health. My life has been one healing lesson after another and I hope that this book will be of value to others who are on the same journey of self-healing and Physical Immortality. I have learned that all illness - even death - are conditions that human beings have created for one reason or another. My healing journey has led me closer to understanding the source of these conditions.

Insomnia

After my father died, I left for my freshman year in college. I was determined to take pre-med and become a nurse, and I was determined to make straight A's. I had a scholarship to Augustana College, a Church college in Sioux Falls, South Dakota. At Augustana, we students had to attend service at the chapel every-day. But all I could do was stand outside the chapel and cry. And I could not sleep. I was afraid to shut my eyes - afraid that I would wake up dead. I really believed that I would die in my sleep. I simply did not sleep. I rarely told anyone about my condition. No one would have believed it anyway, because I was still managing to get straight A's. I was always trying to prove myself. It all took its toll, finally, when I began to have high fevers. I was put in a local hospital and the college called my mother. The doctors told her that they could not find anything wrong with me whatsoever. Once again, I seemed to be manifesting another psychosomatic illness. (Later, I would find out that all illness is *mental* illness.) The doctors asked both her and me if we were willing for me to go into therapy. I had one therapy session with a psychiatrist who put me under hypnosis. After the session, he informed both my mother and me that I was not disturbed enough to warrant his high fees. Bless his honest heart! He suggested that I might need group therapy to share with other people my feelings about my father's death. (Had my cats been with me, I surely would have been OK.)

So I went to group therapy. I was doing okay with it for a while until one of the men there, a minister's son, asked me out for a date. He took me to the movie *Suddenly Last Summer* starring Elizabeth Taylor. Tennessee Williams is pretty intense and, during the movie, I noticed that my date was gripping the arms of the seat as if he were flipping out. When the movie was over, he informed me that he was going back in to see it again, and he left me standing there alone. So much for my first date in college. The next day he was admitted to a psychiatric ward! I went to see him and his father, the minister, was there. "So much for religion," I thought. Religion had failed again and I was really confused.

That summer I worked as a waitress at the Stanley Hotel in Estes Park, Colorado. Keeping busy and serving others healed me. Apparently, there had been 4,000 applications submitted by college students and only thirty were hired by the hotel. I had not even filled out an application. I got the personnel staff's attention by sending them a letter with an explanation of why I thought they should hire me. Even though I was an emotional mess, my higher self was working. (Who wants to sort through 4,000 applications?) Once I started to have fun and became more comfortable with sharing my feelings, I quickly got over insomnia.

Amoebic Dysentery and Acute Cystitis

I finally rebelled and left the Church school and went off to the University of Florida College of Nursing. I went there for two reasons: First, I could get longer summers off which allowed me to work to pay college expenses. Second, it was the second biggest party school in the nation, according to *Playboy Magazine*. I was fed up with the religious and medical dogma of the Midwest. I needed to relax and have some fun! To be able to attend classes in Bermuda shorts and thongs was mind-blowing. I felt that I had experienced a miracle in my life. In a short time, I met a young man who became my husband, a real genius and adventurer. He was an atheist, which was perfect for me. I did not understand the dynamics of it all then, but I was angry with God about my father's long illness and death. I was in love and we married right after my graduation. We were both inspired by President Kennedy to join the Peace Corps. You could say that it was my boot-camp training into world service. Our first assignment was Peru. I was very happy, and we both felt that we were rebelling against the established norms and making a real difference in the world at the same time. It was a dream come true - to travel and serve others.

We had a tough assignment: Chimbote, Peru. It had almost never rained there in modern history. There were squatter settlements everywhere - and no bathrooms! Our hut had no roof per se, only a makeshift pole-and-straw cover. There was no electricity and no running water. People went to the bathroom right in front of everyone else, right in the street. It did not bother me that much to see men peeing in the streets in front of our hut, but to see them with their pants pulled down, squatting, was another thing. At least the women were covered by their long skirts. Just to cook healthful meals was an ordeal. I had to pressure cook everything on the primus stove. It was a real adventure, for sure, and I was determined to see it through.

Before long, we both developed amoebic dysentery despite our preventive efforts. We used to lie in bed and analyze which of us had the worst cramps and which had the most diarrhea. Even though we had been prepared for the possibility of this illness, blood in our stools was a scary thing, even for a nurse. Eventually, my husband lost his hair. He had developed a much rarer and stronger form of the amoeba.

What I was not prepared for was an acute attack of severe pain in my kidneys and blood in my urine. It was like urinating razor blades. I recognized the symptoms from my nursing books: honeymoon cystitis. It was excruciating. One did not dare consider going to a hospital in that town. The beds had no sheets and there was filth everywhere. I had been taking care of babies in that hospital in the worst conditions, and I had seen many babies die of illness and starvation. Plague epidemics were on the rise and my husband wired Lima. A Peace Corps helicopter came to evacuate me out of there.

Somehow the word got out that I was really sick. I did not think I was so sick at the time. I thought that I had IVS and that I was going to be fine. Many of the Peace Corps volunteers heard that I was dying and left their posts to visit me. Despite the rumors, I recovered for the time being; but the condition continued and became more chronic later on. Many times during my marriage, it got so bad that I ended up hospitalized, needing dilation and other treatments. Sometimes I had to stay on Macrodantin for a year at a time. I became afraid of sex. It ruined my and my husband's sex life. The medical profession could not cure me of this condition. I was a nurse in those days and I had no idea of alternative healing methods.

My husband and I ended up getting a divorce and I began to have fewer problems with cystitis and more sexual experience. What was it about my husband? I know now that I had not experienced any form of enlightenment during my marriage because I was stuck in conventional medical concepts. Also, I knew nothing about the ideas of past lives and karma. The whole experience remained a mystery to me until I realized that I developed cystitis only with certain types of men.

Then, one day I met Leonard Orr and I learned about Rebirthing. I became more conscious of the metaphysical and I started getting serious about alternative healing. It was not until I had experienced several LRT's that I was able to crack the cystitis case completely.

Once, before a training session in Boston, I had a

very frightening dream that five men came into my room and left a tarantula on my bed. I woke, terrified and screaming. The next morning at the coffee shop, five men came in and sat down with me at my table. I panicked and tried to remain calm. During the sex therapy section of the training, I nearly fainted. Fortunately, my trainer kept going with the session. I pulled out a piece of paper and did some automatic writing: "Five men, rape, Africa". After that I was on the floor in a spontaneous Rebirthing.

Was my ex-husband one of those men? Some alternative healers have found that, when we are younger, we often are attracted to past-life mates with whom we have karmic experiences to balance out. We have to do this before we can move on to more loving and whole relationships. The next day after the session in Boston, I happened to have an appointment with a famous aura reader. She told me that I had almost totally worked out that karma. Prior to that I had never understood how past-life experience could come back to inflict our bodies. I had healed from the cystitis though. *It was a matter of bringing up the cause and letting it go!*

14 Years of Migrating Pain

In addition to insomnia, after my father died, I began to experience a lot of physical pain in my body. This condition developed right after I saw my father in his casket. The pains were intense at times and they migrated around my body. The whole experience was very unusual to me because, prior to my father's dying, I had had no pains. I realized that it was all psychosomatic and I knew that "doctors" could not help me. I learned to live with those pains for fourteen years until I began Rebirthing. After three sessions, the mysterious pains left my body and never returned. It was a question of breathing out the "death urge" that had been taken in from my family and activated in me. Now you can understand why I became a Rebirther!

Severe Hair Loss

My hair had always been naturally curly. In fact, it had gotten so curly while I was in Florida that I bought some hair straightener and almost ruined my hair. But that was nothing compared to what happened to my hair after my divorce. It began falling out, to the point that I had a large bald spot and I had to wear a wig to hide it. The more worried I got, the more hair I lost. I was a nurse and had access to the best doctors. I went to so many that it became ridiculous. None of them could help me. I was in constant therapy, but that did not help me either. I was desperate and I was really scared. This all happened prior to my first Rebirthing experience and prior to my metaphysical awakening. I was still deeply entrenched in the "modern" medical approach to healing. Nothing was working for me and I became suicidal, which made it even worse.

One day in Phoenix, I visited yet one more dermatologist. I had decided that he would be the final one. He had white hair and was a sweet "father figure". I trusted him. He suggested that I save the amount of hair that fell out each week and put it into a sack and bring it in to him. He wanted to study the amounts to determine if they were increasing or decreasing. It was always increasing, and the sacks got fuller.

One week he looked at me and said, "My dear, you have a very serious problem".

"You're telling me!" I shrieked. "You are my last hope. I cannot stand to go to another doctor."

Well, he went to his prescription book and wrote down the following:

GO READ THIS BOOK: *Peace of Mind*
by Rabbi Leiberman

I was shocked. "What kind of prescription was this?" I wondered. I read the book and was blown away. It was my first real exposure to metaphysical philosophy. It explained how the mind rules the body. Why had not any of the nursing books that I had studied covered this? I will always be grateful to the man. My hair stopped falling out, but I still had quite a bald spot. I was going into my third year with this condition.

I remember looking into the mirror and saying, "What if this never ends?" I had to deal with this fear every single day. But, after one straight year of Rebirthing, I worked out almost all of the tension that was preventing my hair from becoming healthy. I had some help at that time from my friend, Dr. Irv Katz. He did a couple of hypnotic sessions with me. I really trusted him for he was a fellow Rebirther, LRT graduate, sex therapist and a great psychologist. He got me right down to all my unconscious issues of loss. Between the Rebirthing and the sessions with Dr. Katz, I was healed. My hair grew back! It was a miracle for me, and my friends could not believe it. I went on a marvelous trip to Hawaii and was finally free of that condition. The whole experience was a powerful lesson for me.

Isn't it amazing how the issues of loss from my childhood manifested into a real, physical condition of loss in my body? My mind, conscious or unconscious, really did rule my body!

Food Neurosis

I was born on the kitchen table, so maybe my food neurosis started then. My birth trauma was all wired up with food. In one of my past-life regression experiences, I found out that I had been poisoned by some food. Maybe it all started then. I was always neurotic about food, even as a child. I was terrified about getting fat and I ate like a bird. To gain even five pounds extra drove me insane. It was my own private and inner hell.

My mother was a home economics teacher and we lived in the heart of the Midwest where most of the nation's food is grown. Everyone at home was obsessed with food. Well, it seemed that way to me, anyway: In the morning, you get up, think about breakfast, prepare breakfast, eat breakfast and then clean up after breakfast. Then you think about lunch, prepare lunch, eat lunch and then clean up after lunch.

You go through the whole cycle for dinner and even the bedtime snack. My mother was always concerned with food - what you eat with what. The only fights we ever had were in the kitchen and were about food - what to cook or how to prepare it. And then there was the fact that my father took twelve different pills at every single meal. He used to lay them all out on his plate. This always reminded me of his illness and that he might be dying. I wanted to get out of there and out of the obsession with food.

At one point in my life, I got so neurotic about eating that I actually began to fear eating off my own plate. This got especially intense when my past-life stuff was coming up. I became increasingly paranoid and would have to eat off one of my friends' plates. Fortunately, most of my friends were very understanding. They would tell me to take a walk around the block or something which would help me get a grip on myself.

In the late seventies, my neurosis came to a head while visiting my guru, Babaji, in India. Once, in his presence, I became very nervous and obsessed with the subject of food. I was not overweight at all but I was constantly worried about it. I lived on the edge of anorexia all the time, but it was ridiculous for me to be experiencing those fears in Babaji's ashram. I decided to confess my obsession to him for I was, literally, on the verge of severe neurosis. One day I walked right up to him and said, " Babaji, I am totally obsessed and neurotic about the topic of food."

He looked at me and abruptly said, "Oh, just give up food," and then he walked away.

I took this very seriously. Was he implying that I should become a Breatharian and be like Saint Teresa Newman who ate only one communion wafer a day for 25 years? I went back to Babaji and asked him if he meant right now.

"No," he said, "the food here is holy and blessed. You give up food when you go back to America."

I was still a neophyte around Babaji. I took everything that he said literally. I did not understand his ways, his methods or his lilas: divine tricks or playing of the Master to help you crack your problems. What followed then was really difficult. I began to go nuts and I tried to imagine never eating again. I was not a vegetarian at the time, and I began to have visions of sizzling steaks going by right in the temple and in the presence of Babaji. Then I would see large pizzas, dripping with cheese. These visions were in vivid color and kept getting stronger. I could no longer pray, chant or meditate. I was losing my mind.

Finally, one evening, I knelt before Babaji and once again told the truth: "I've gone crazy now."

Suddenly, he picked up two large cymbals...the kind that one would see in a marching band. He raised them up over my head and crashed them together as hard as he could. My body shook wildly and then it was over. My mind cleared completely. Babaji had given me some type of "sound healing". Later, I realized that I had never seen those cymbals around him before that moment, nor did I see them any time thereafter. Had he materialized a set of symbols for my healing? Was it all a dream?

And yet, still taking Babaji literally, when I left India

I gave up food as he had told me to do. He had also told
me to walk every morning at 4 a.m. I was in Hawaii and
I gave up food for thirty days. Every morning I got up
and walked. I was not hungry but I felt really angry. I
would have to take long walks to clear the anger. After
thirty days of this routine, I realized that it was all just a
lila (divine play) and the whole point of it all was for me
to process some of my anger about death. I started to
feel better and eat normally.

There were a few setbacks, though. I was fine until
some of my friends and I piled into a car and drove to
Mexico for a lobster feed. We were on a beach with
Mariachis playing and unlimited amounts of lobster
that just kept coming and coming. I wondered how my
friends could eat so much and still be so happy. I
reached my limit right away and then all my fear came
up again. On the way home from that trip, I curled up
in the fetal position and prayed to Babaji and Jesus for
liberation. I pleaded once again for help. Then I heard
the words, *"The Only Diet There Is"*, and I realized that
I was being told to write another book.

Other than this book, that book was the hardest one
I ever wrote. One third of the way through I got severe
writer's block and could not write anything for a year. I
was really struggling. But, thanks to my friend, R.R.,
who was a brilliant restaurateur, I broke through. He
could eat any amount of food without gaining weight
or getting full. I picked his brain and his secrets
worked. I dedicated that book to him. I was able to
finally break through my writer's block and my food
neurosis condition - and I was able to finish the book. It
was that chapter on *The Ego and Food* that I really put it

all together. Afterwards, it did not matter what I ate and I stopped thinking about the whole issue. I had always wanted to be able to eat anything and not gain weight. By the time I finally achieved that, I was bored with food altogether. I was finally liberated. It felt like heaven to be free of that ridiculous pattern.

Acute Arthritis

All of my healing issues were beginning to dissolve as I came deeper into metaphysical understanding. I was beginning to feel really good. It was a thrill to be at the beginning of Rebirthing and studying with Leonard Orr. I was over my divorce, had a new boyfriend and we were in San Francisco during the heyday of the alternative consciousness movement. We were living in a spiritual community, and Leonard Orr was teaching us the concepts of Physical Immortality. I had already been working out my unconscious death urge the hard way, so I adapted quickly to Leonard's ideas. I wanted to live and I wanted to be healthy. I was ecstatic to learn that I may be able to prolong my life. I gave up nursing and "modern" medicine that year. One day I just walked out. Why should I stay in a profession that was not producing the quick and Permanent Healings that I was seeing in Rebirthing? (See page 155 on *Rebirthing and Healing*)

I was so enthusiastic about Rebirthing that I told Leonard that I thought I should write a book for Rebirthers and include all the information on Physical Immortality. Most of that information was underground and I was beginning to dig it out. I felt that my second book should be called *Rebirthing in the New Age*. I wanted to write it with Leonard and I told him that we needed a chapter on Physical Immortality. That night we tossed the I Ching to see if the world was ready for such a book. The I Ching came out with the following; "Yes, but you are on very thin ice." We decided to write it.

I locked myself in seclusion and began the chapter on Immortality. I had no idea how much would come up from my subconscious mind. I was in a bit over my head. It was still a very radical thing to talk about these subjects. Then, a few days into it, my fingers locked up with gripping pain. I ran into Leonard's room crying hysterically.

"Leonard," I shouted, "I have arthritis!" I knew I could have a brilliant writing career and I was barely getting started. Now it might all be over!

He looked at me calmly and said, "Oh, this is great!"

"What do you mean?" I screamed at him, "How can this be great?"

Then he said that it was because I was going through my old age early and that he did not have to worry about me anymore. He was not concerned at all. I began to relax. Only an Immortal could have gotten me through that moment. I began Rebirthing feverishly for three weeks to process out the arthritis. It worked! Rebirthing had healed me again.

The important thing that I learned is that we need to be in the presence of enlightened friends who do not go into agreement with our negative conditions. If Leonard had gotten as upset as I had, I would have been sunk and, most likely, would have arthritis to this day. This is exactly how Jesus healed people. He never affirmed their egos. He only saw them healed. I went through several early aging releases after this.

Leonard Orr once said, "It is better to go through that stuff when you are young and strong enough to really process it."

Severe Sinusitis

I was in Bali with close associates and friends. We were all having a great time and it was my birthday. That afternoon, I developed a sudden sinus block without any warning. I had not been sick for a long time and I thought that it would just pass. It did not pass, and later I realized that it had started the exact time of my birth: 2:30 in the afternoon, August 24th. It took me a while to put the connection together. I continued to travel and the condition kept getting worse, especially with the flying. I went from healer to healer and worked on myself constantly. By then I had learned how to clear my mind much better, but it was not working on my sinus infection. Nothing I did helped, nor were the healers I visited able to clear the problem. When it finally sunk in, that the condition really had started at the exact time of my birth, I called Dr. Bob Doughten, the only obstetrician I knew in the States that was also a Rebirther. He had actually been Rebirthing teenagers whom he had delivered years before! That really impressed me and I was anxious to see him.

I flew to Portland where he lived and I suggested that he Rebirth me on the kitchen floor since I was born in the kitchen. He was more than willing. It is great to have a good Rebirther, but it is the ultimate to have an obstetrician to Rebirth you! Wow! There is nothing like that! I told him that I thought I needed to review my whole birth one more time. I asked him to imagine pulling me out. He put his hands on my head when I was breathing. Then he suddenly said, "Oh, I see they pulled you out wrong."

I felt pain around my nose and shouted, "I am damaged!" and I re-experienced my sinus area being nearly crushed by the doctor who actually delivered me.

I had stopped the birth process myself, waiting for my father to come back into the kitchen. He had gone out to the porch to light a cigarette!!! That is when the doctor tried to pull me out. I had wanted to wait a little longer. (Cigarettes had affected my whole life!) I remembered the whole scenario then and there.

Dr. Doughten sat me up, looked into my eyes and said, "You know that you have the power to heal this yourself but you are not doing it. You are setting your life up in such a way that you have to go back to 'modern' medicine so that you are forced to forgive doctors."

I knew that he was right. Large tears flew out from my eyes towards his eyes and I promised him that I would go.

In Denver, I opened the phone book to Professional Specialists in ENT. I ran my finger down the page and it stopped at Dr. Roy Jones. The only appointment that I could get was at 2:30 in the afternoon, the exact time of my birth! I walked into his office and almost fell over. He looked exactly like Dr. Moore, my obstetrician! I couldn't believe it. I was thinking that it all had to be a Babaji lila, and I told my assistant, Wendy, to help me surrender to this doctor totally. I was not going to fight anything that he said.

When he came back with the X-rays, he said, "These are Opaque Four. I cannot possibly let you leave here without surgery! You must avoid all flying and you are very lucky that you don't have optic nerve damage. I just cannot believe that you have been walking around with this condition."

So there it was. Did I dare confess to him my arrogance...that I thought I would never need a doctor again and that I had no insurance? He was very kind and understanding when I told him the truth. He arranged it so that I could go in as an outpatient and go right home after the surgery.

The last thing that I ever wanted to do was to go back to "modern" medicine, but I remembered what Dr. Bob Doughten had said and I humbled myself. The whole ordeal turned into a very spiritual experience. The nurses had somehow read my books. They were like angels. The surgeon introduced me to the anesthesiologist saying that they had an excellent relationship and had gone to school together. While I was in the waiting room, the surgeon came out and called my name. He said that my surgery went very well!

I thought I was losing it for a moment and said, "Wait a minute, I have not even gone in yet!"

He seemed confused and ruffled. Was he channeling my name or the outcome of the as yet unperformed surgery? I took it as a message from Babaji that everything was going to be okay. I went into the operating room relaxed. Apparently, while under anesthesia, I gave everyone in the room a very clear lecture on how dolphins were programmed by Atlanteans. They were all amazed and I hear they still talk about it.

Later, I visited a healer in Madrid who was very strong but said very little. I had told him nothing about my ordeal. He passed his hand over my sinus area and said only, "Karmic break".

Then I saw that I had allowed myself to be experimented upon with some type of lasers in ancient Atlantis...something to do with the uplifting of humanity. (I could imagine myself doing that!)

The whole experience of severe sinusitis taught me that many, if not all, of our physical conditions are absolutely linked to our past. Whether it be past lives, birth traumas or childhood conditioning, our illnesses and physical problems are almost always rooted in some form of negative, unconscious memory that can be discovered and released through Rebirthing and other methods of alternative healing.

Acute Hypothermia

I took time off from my own healing journey and went home to see my sister shortly before she died of melanoma. Her aura was very gray and she was very angry. I spent hours with her while she vented her feelings. I tried to help her as much as I could. I gave her lists of people who had healed themselves of cancer. I gave her lists of healers who had actually been successful healing people with cancer. I was hoping that she would ask for help - but to no avail.

She had not even read my books! I was a heretic in her eyes. When she flat-out refused to read the lists, I was devastated.

When I left her that last time, I began to experience intense cold and freezing chills throughout my body. Apparently, I was channeling through me as much of my family's death urge as I could stand which triggered more of my own. I shook and shook. I could not get warm, no matter what I did. The cold got so intense that, when I walked into a room, the heat from the venting systems would turn cold and the hot water in the taps would do the same. It happened several times...even in my friend Fred's room. He was a personal witness to this bizarre phenomena.

I could not shake the chills. Even when I was wearing a warm coat at the airports, people would walk up to me and tell me that I looked cold! Finally, I decided that a trip to the hot springs in California was in order. By a small miracle, I attracted a polarity therapist who was able to teach me how to treat my condition. He told me to stay in the hot water as long as I could stand it and then to go directly into cold water. I could not imagine going into cold water, but he said that it would "set the heat" in my bones. I followed his instructions and it worked. I was able connect with Mother Nature and heal through another bout with that old death urge.

Melanoma

About six months after my sister died, I was in New Delhi with my then boyfriend. He was a yogi

who had spent about ten years in India. Before that he
had been a "doctor". By the grace of Babaji, he was
there with me. He happened to notice a mole on my
left leg and told me that it was serious and needed to
be taken out. I had not even noticed anything wrong.
It looked like an ordinary mole to me. I was working
hard to tune out illness and my past connections with
ordinary "medicine" - not dwell on them. I could tell
that he was channeling and I figured I had better listen
to him. When we were back in the States, I went to
get it checked. Sure enough, it was melanoma. I was
shocked. I was not the cancer type at all. Was I going
into sympathy with my sister? Was it my last ditch
approach to win her love by being like her and manifesting the same death stuff?

   It turned out that the melanoma was not very deep
and they were able to get it all.

   Exactly one year after my sister's death, I was in
Atlanta.   I went into a major death trauma or some-
thing and threw myself on the bed while screaming,
"I want to live! I want to live!"

   I called my friend Rhonda to help me. For four days
I went through intense paranoia about dying and I did
not want to be alone. There was nothing wrong with
me physically whatsoever. Rhonda's son was there and
he had happened to cut himself and needed to see a
doctor. I went with them and mentioned my fear condition to the doctor.

   When I told him that it had been exactly one year
since my sister had died, he asked me, "Don't you
know that it is very common for family members to
have strong delayed reactions one year after a loved

one's death?" Somehow his words cleared me.

Later, I was in Bali again and I was having a wonderful time. But one night I woke up having a horrible nightmare. I saw my sister and she was deranged. I woke up screaming and saw that another spot of skin cancer had popped up overnight on my leg! I was confused and could not understand what was going on. I went to my altar and started praying. I was not about to go to a doctor in Indonesia. My next stop on the trip was India. There I went to see a doctor who was a Babaji devotee. He looked up at the pictures of our Guru and said, "Let's see what the Old Master has in store for you."

Later, he called the chief surgeon of Delhi who had treated the President of India. That doctor was one of the best available and had studied in London. Okay, I could handle that. The clinic was marginal, but I trusted him. He told me that I needed to have it out quickly just in case it was malignant. I was not going to mess around with melanoma. That form of cancer could move very fast. I decided to go ahead with the surgery and process my mind later.

Fortunately, I was on my way to Rajistan to see my guru Shastriji. I cried at his feet and begged him to explain what was going on with me. What he said to me then gave me the shock of my life.

He said, "I regret to tell you, but your sister has not crossed over properly. She has been entering your body to get attention because she knows that you are the only one advanced enough to help her."

"What?" I said, "How could this be?" These weird things could not possibly happen to MY family. "Is he talking about possession?" I wondered.

He told me that I had to follow his instructions exactly and that, if it didn't work, I would have to go to the Banares - the place where souls cross over. Banares... I could not believe it! Shastriji also told me that I had to immediately chant 5,000 mantras for her and perform a fire ceremony. Then I would have to perform a ceremony for all the dead in the Ganges and wait to see if my sister would appear to me again. I did exactly what my guru instructed but, let me tell you, it was one of the hardest tasks in my life.

I had never tried 5,000 mantras before. I did 1,000 a day for five days. I focused almost all my attention toward my sister. While in Delhi, I became terrified at the thought of not being able to complete what Shastriji had instructed me to do to help my sister. What if her soul were lost in the cosmos for thousands of years? I got really scared and cried for hours. At one point, I was so upset that I had to go next door to the hotel room of my friends, Carmen and Adolfo. I got in bed with the whole family. They held me while I worked on my breathing. Adolfo was my perfect Rebirther. He shared with me how his brother had died in his arms from an overdose of drugs.

My "group", which consisted of students coming from all over the world to train with me in India, was about to arrive at the hotel at any time. I had to recover! I put all my soul into that Rebirthing, finished my mantras, and all the fear cleared just five minutes before I had to go down and meet my students. Later, I performed the ceremonies just as Shastriji had instructed. My sister appeared to me. She seemed all right. I obviously had something to work out and clear with her in order to stop manifesting cancer in my body. I went to a few past-life therapists and reviewed all my karma with my sister. I received amazing information. If I had not worked all of that through and released it, I surely would have struggled with more bouts of cancer over and over. As of today, I have been completely healed of melanoma!

After that ordeal, I found peace with my issues about "modern" medicine. Many times, people have a lot of fear about self-healing, and must therefore rely on doctors for help. Self-healing can be a very deep and complicated issue and we all need help to make the gradual transition to alternative healing methods. But I have found that prayer helps and that, through prayer, we can always attract the perfect healers in our lives when we need them.

Rheumatism

After my first experience of writing a chapter on Physical Immortality (when I got arthritis), I was terrified of the prospect of writing a whole book on the subject. It took me nine years to get up the courage. I did not have a computer in those days. When I finally decided it was time to tackle this project, I bought a new electric typewriter. To my dismay, the typewriter kept blowing up and I had to keep taking it back.

"Ma'am," the man at the store said, "You're too powerful...you have to upgrade."

I had to keep upgrading until I ended up with absolutely the most expensive model they had (of course). But then the lights in my flat started blowing out and a lot of strange things began to happen. I was busy writing and I didn't let it bother me that much. It felt as though there were other forces at work around me and coming through me. There was a force of resistance as well but, somehow, I got through it.

When I called my mother to tell her that I had written the most important manuscript of my life, I was so happy and *alive.* It was during that same phone call that I first found out about my sister's cancer. All of the joy I had been feeling drained out of me immediately. Shortly afterward, the book was released. I remember when I saw the first hardback edition: I was signing books in Los Angeles and the line for autographs was longer than I had ever experienced. As the line finally got towards the end, I felt a very strange "reaction" in my body. Suddenly, I felt extremely odd and as heavy as lead.

The next morning I was preparing to give a speech on the subject of Physical Immortality at a local Los Angeles church. While I was dressing, I suddenly experienced the sensation of shattering glass in my left hip and I fell to the floor. The pain was terrible. I crawled to the phone and called a friend who was an excellent psychic. I pleaded with him to tell me what was happening. He said that the topic of my presentation was opposed to that which the church usually teaches and that I was meeting some real resistance. I told him that I was going despite whatever was blocking me. I cried in the taxi all the way to the church. There was no doubt that I was having a spontaneous Rebirthing.

When I arrived at the church, I immediately told the staff that I needed to lie down. "How much time do I have?" I asked.

"Twenty minutes...and the only place to lie down would be in the kitchen," someone said. This was perfect, of course, for I was born in the kitchen!

Some of the Rebirthers in the audience saw me coming in, realized that I was in trouble and got up to help me. I was crying and breathing like mad trying to get ready for my talk, but the time ran out. Someone opened the swinging door and shouted, "You're on!"

My eye makeup was running down my face, my suit was wrinkled, and I could hardly walk. My body felt like old age was setting in and fast. It was clear to me that I had developed the symptoms of rheumatism. I had to be helped all the way to the stage. I was a mess and hardly in any kind of shape to give a lecture on *How to be Chic and Fabulous.* I told the audience that I had to go through this in front of them. People started crying in the audience and some of them went into spontaneous Rebirthing right there. Imagine their meeting me for the first time while I was in that condition!

Suddenly, my energy shifted and I gave a brilliant lecture on *The Immortals of the Bible.* I don't remember any of it except the fact that I was given a standing ovation. After that, I was right back on the kitchen floor in pain. I stayed most of the afternoon on a couch unable to move.

I remembered that someone had put a phone number of an acupuncturist whom they liked in my coat pocket. That was one of the little miracles that has kept me going as a public figure. I went for a treatment and it helped me a lot. At least I was able to get on my feet and walk. But, for the next few days, when I visited my Rebirthing clients in Hollywood, I had to hobble up to those mansions like a little old lady. It was really embarrassing. On top of it all, I had to go to Australia in that condition. For three whole weeks I had severe symptoms of rheumatism. I had chiropractic treatments and all kinds of other treatments. When I got back to the States, I called my mother to ask her how she was.

"Oh," she said, "I had a real bad spell with my hip these past weeks but now it's gone."

Later that day, my hip suddenly healed and I have not had the problem since. What was it with my family and me? Was my health that psychically connected to theirs? Was this their stuff or mine?

After that experience, I became really confused about all my strange physical conditions and about my sensitivity to other people's illness and death. I knew that Babaji could process other people's stuff and worlds of karma through his body all the time, but he knew how to do it. I was obviously not very good at it. I began to wonder where the boundaries of my being were.

Gastritis

I was working in Berlin. It was shortly after the Wall came down. I was very sensitive to all the personal and social trauma that surrounded it all. It so happened that my two nieces were in Germany and my mother was coming to visit all of us. There we were, meeting together for the first time since my sister had died. I found out for the first time that my niece had been pregnant when her mother (my sister) passed on. The baby had been born with disabilities. We were all emotional wrecks and it was all just too much for me. I could not digest it and I could not digest Berlin. Out of nowhere I developed a terrible pain in my upper intestines. I could not eat and I wondered if I had manifested an ulcer.

Like so many times before, I was privileged to have a wonderful assistant who was actually an obstetrician. She was amazing - also a trained Rebirther and a rock star! She was fun to be around and she cheered me up.

For the first time in quite a while, I had a chance to really talk with my mother. I asked her if I had suffered with colic or something as an infant.

To my shock, she said, "Yes...for six weeks."

I asked her why I had colic and she said, "Oh, some babies have colic and some don't."

That answer did not satisfy me at all. I told her that it had probably been caused by the cow's milk and that I thought that I was angry that she had not breast-fed me. She was understanding and agreed that maybe I was right.

Later, I asked my assistant-Rebirther to give me a deep session on the issue of breast-feeding. I went back to the time of my infancy and found that I had feelings and pre-verbal thoughts that translated to something like this: "I can never forgive this! They might as well put me out in the street!" I was really angry that I had not been breast-fed. No wonder I had suffered with colic as an infant and no wonder that I had developed gastritis as an adult.

I started to pray very hard to Babaji. I cried at my altar and pleaded with him to help me. I wondered how I was going to do a whole European tour when I could not even eat. Then, a miracle happened. I was doing the seminar with mostly all German people. An Italian man walked in late. I could not understand what he was doing there and I wondered if he could understand English or the German translation.

At the break, we ended up in the same elevator and he introduced himself as Michaelangelo.

I suddenly blurted out, "Oh, you are the one for Italy. Please come to my room after we finish." I was startled at myself for being so direct. The words had just come out of my mouth but I had learned before to trust these things. He seemed to have no problem with it at all.

Later, he came to my room. He was a divine being and an angel. Then, to my amazement, he told me that he was a devotee of Babaji and Muniraj. I was astonished. He told me that he had been "called" to come, that he had actually been in a car wreck on the way, but felt that he still had to make it to the seminar. It turned out to be another Babaji miracle for me. I felt compelled to tell him about my condition and he said that he could help. He pulled some very fine, high-vibration food out of his bag. It looked like vegetable pate and baby food. He fed me as if I were an infant and I was able to eat a little. My prayers had been answered.

He told me that he could heal me in two weeks if I could travel to Milan. It was a nice idea but I had a whole tour to complete and I could not arrange to get away. The rest of the trip, I managed to eat a teaspoon of bee pollen each day and a few fresh dates while in Spain. I was not able to eat anything else, literally.

During this period, many people began telling me that I needed to take time off. That was the last thing I wanted to hear. I was a workaholic who could not stop. But then a funny thing happened: Perfect strangers started walking up to me on the streets and telling me that I needed to take time off. This happened so many times that I realized it must Babaji speaking to me through other people and that I had better wake up.

I canceled part of my tours and rented a cottage on Cape Cod. Then I sent Michaelangelo a plane ticket for he had agreed to come and stay with me for a few weeks. The day before he came, I decided that I would ask him to shave my head. I was in trouble with my body, and I wanted to facilitate the maximum healing possible in the manner that I had learned from my gurus in India. I called my mother to tell her how happy I was with my decision. I had done this before, so I thought that she could handle it this time. She was not happy at all. It was the one thing about my spiritual journey that was just too much for her. Besides, she had made plans for me to visit relatives and she didn't think it would be good for them to see me that way. I told her I just would not go and that my healing would have to take top priority. It was hard, but it was all I could do. I knew that she would get over it in time. Would I ever get over my stomach condition if I did not take some time for myself? I wanted to be in optimum cooperation with whatever Michaelangelo wanted to do. I had to surrender.

I prepared an altar in my cottage. Then I fixed up a

basket with all the necessities for the head-shave (mundun). I covered the basket with a sacred cloth and put it under the altar. I even called an astrologer to ask when the perfect time would be. She was astonished that the time I had chosen was absolutely perfect - Fourth of July and she suggested one minute before midnight.

That night, one of my students picked up Michael-angelo at the airport and drove him to my cottage. It was good to see him. I immediately told him about my desire and he was agreeable to the idea. He had abso-lutely no problem accepting the sacred responsibility. After all, he had had his head shaved several times, and he understood the deep meaning and power this type of healing gives.

We started the mundun one minute before midnight. It took quite a while and I was awake all night. I had shaved my head twice before and I thought that a third time would be a snap. But I was shocked at how spiritually strong it was. I lay on the couch for days feeling my energy chakras swirling around and around. It was a very strange sensation and I felt as though I were turning inside out.

Michaelangelo began giving me an hour and a half session of reflexology twice a day. He is a master and his touch was very intense. He also prepared and fed me his high-vibration foods each day. It was hard for me to digest even little amounts, but I managed to get down small portions. After about ten days, I began to have a real healing crisis and started to go kind of berserk. He helped me by taking me for long walks and making me walk faster and faster. That got my breathing into a constant Rebirthing mode. The final week he took some time to go to one of my LRTs in Connecticut. It was my gift to him. When he came back, he was excited, but had gone through an energy shift himself. He ended up on the floor, breathing and Rebirthing through his own healing crisis before he went back to Italy!

By the end of his visit, I was much better. I left Cape Cod and went to Bali for a rest. It was wonderful to be on that island and with a shaved head! I was so glad that I had taken some time for self-healing and I was so grateful to Michaelangelo.

After Bali, I went to India. I wanted to give my thanks and prayers to Babaji. While I was in the Himalayas, I met a beautiful Dutch man. We really hit it off and both felt that we had been together in a past life as young lovers in Poland. Well, it just so happened that I was scheduled to do the first ever LRT given in Poland right after my mission in India. Naturally, my new friend decided to travel with me.

The whole experience of gastritis taught me that an adult healing crisis is often directly related to a childhood or infancy crisis. In my case, I was able to bring up my feelings of lack and anger at not being breast-fed and deal with them. I was able to let them go and receive some special healing before they ate a hole in my body. The symptom is not the illness nor is it the problem. The source of healing is much deeper and related to the condition of our mental and emotional selves. I can only be eternally grateful that I was able to expand my awareness beyond "modern" medicine and traditional religion.

The Basics of Metaphysical Healing

* The mind rules the body.

* The body is the effect of the mind.

* Negative thoughts produce negative results in the body.

* What you think expands in the material-physical world.

* Anything can be cured. We create illness with our minds and we can *uncreate* it with our minds.

* We will give up pain or the symptom when we see no more value in it. *(Course in Miracles)*

* The real physician is the mind of the patient. The outcome of healing is what the mind of the patient decides. *(Course in Miracles)*

* Disease is often anger taken out on the body.

* It is an immutable spiritual law that when there is a health problem, there is a forgiveness problem. (Catherine Ponder, *Dynamic Laws of Healing*)

* You have healing power within you. *Permanent Healing* comes from freeing the mind and health is basically an inside job. The mind is in every cell of your body. Every cell is enveloped in thought. Your body is composed of radiant substance. The body is soft, pliable and even plastic to your thoughts.
(Catherine Ponder)

* All healing is, essentially, the release from fear. Fear causes pain and disease.

* Resentment, anger, hate, condemnation and the desire to get even will tear down your body.

* You are not a victim. There are no victims. Life presents to us whatever our thoughts are...conscious or unconscious.

Part II

Causes of Sickness

"There is nothing that is incurable except that which you acknowledge as incurable."

"To change your body, all that you have to do is change your mind and your body will change automatically."

Leonard Orr
Founder of Rebirthing

Negative Thoughts and Personal Lies

PERSONAL LIES CAN MAKE YOU SICK AND KEEP
YOU FROM HEALING YOURSELF!

In my other books I have often discussed how our
most negative thoughts can affect our lives. These
include negative, pre-verbal thoughts from birth and
infancy. In this chapter, I will try to show you how
these negative thoughts can sabotage our ability to heal
ourselves. A personal law or "lie" is our most negative
thought about ourselves, usually formed at birth, in the
womb, or brought in as a core belief from a past life.
Originally, we called these thoughts "personal laws"
because we believe them to be true and they can control
our whole lives. But since it is not the *real* truth about
ourselves, we now emphasize that these thoughts are
"personal lies".

Here are some of the most common "personal lies" that
we have seen in Rebirthing:

I am not good enough
I am bad
I am wrong
I am not perfect
I am weak
I am guilty
I can't
I can't make it
I am a failure

There is something wrong with me
I am a disappointment
I shouldn't be here
I am unwanted
I am evil
I am stuck
I am nothing

In everyone we have Rebirthed, we have been able to find one of the above thoughts predominant. The person's tendency is to act out the negative thought, or to suppress it and over-compensate and/or project it onto someone else. For example, persons with the thought, "I am bad," may go around acting bad and doing things that are bad, bringing on themselves bad judgment from others and actually reinforcing the thought of "badness". Or they may work very hard to keep the thought of being bad completely hidden from other people and overcompensate by acting especially good all the time. They may become obsessed with being good, not seeing their behavior as only a cover-up. Or, finally, they may project their "bad" thought onto others and start seeing everyone else as bad instead of facing such defects in themselves.

Unfortunately, these thoughts are like addictions. A person believes a thought so strongly that, after years and years of accepting it, the thought just seems to be normal. It also feels as though one's life depends almost totally upon keeping that thought alive. The person starts believing that that is who they really are. Having survived both birth and infancy with that thought, the person suffers an unconscious fear that he or she would die if they should give up the thought. Of course, this does not make any sense. It is just a trick of the ego.

Some people mistakenly think that as soon as they discover their "personal lie", they can drop it overnight. Unfortunately, we have found it is not that easy. People usually fear an overnight shift in habit patterns. They fear too much light or too much of an energy change all at once. Most people tend to chip away at the negative thought and let it go slowly over time.

These negative thoughts are in the deep subconscious, so most people might not even be aware that they have a block unless they experience Rebirthing or some similar purification technique. Please let me give an example of how each of these negative thoughts can interfere with healing:

I am not good enough: These people might accept the idea that they are not good enough to be healed. So, no matter how many healing opportunities have been given, none would help because deep down these people believe that they are not good enough to deserve the result of healing. So they will create *The Sabotage Pattern.*

I am bad: These persons usually believe that bad people must be punished and one of the punishments that they deserve is the sickness that they have. Just as in the former case, they are likely to sabotage any healing.

I am wrong: People who think they are wrong will also

think that they deserve punishment, and the illness may be the very punishment they think they deserve. These people may also attract the "wrong" diagnosis, the "wrong" medicine, the "wrong" doctor or healer and never get anywhere. They could even get stuck on working in the wrong part of their mind on the wrong issues.

I am not perfect: These people often make up little things wrong in their bodies so they can feel imperfect. They might be obsessed with the imperfections they create. As soon as they heal one imperfection, they will make up another so they can make sure they are never perfect. Often, they will never be satisfied with the doctor or healer that they choose, projecting that the doctor or healer is imperfect! Even if they should find the perfect doctor or healer, they might set up their treatment so something would go wrong and they could remain imperfect.

I am weak: These people may make up an illness that results in a feeling of weakness. Then they can physically experience the fact that they are weak, thus manifesting the "proof" that they are weak. They might create an ilness like anemia, for example, or Epstein-Barr Syndrome, Chronic Fatigue Syndrome or something else that saps their energy. Often, these people are premature at birth and get stuck in the thought, "I am too weak to heal myself."

I am guilty: Since guilt demands punishment, this person will make sure that he or she is punished somehow. They might become sexually promiscuous so that they can continue the guilt cycle and then end up with a sexually transmitted disease. They may create something like herpes out of healthy, normal sex. They may punish themselves in a number of ways - from losing money, friends, a good job, to anything else that feeds the guilt and causes them to suffer. Of course the most natural way to take out guilt is on the body and these people may create not getting healed because they feel too guilty to deserve healing.

I can't or I can't make it: Sometimes these people create mysterious illnesses or diseases that cannot be diagnosed. They will think that they absolutely can't be healed. Thoughts of helplessness and despair get stretched out to, "I can't let go...I can't get rid of this...I can't control my body." These people can really get stuck in the thought "I can't let go of the thought, I can't." (Not to worry, trained Rebirthers know how to handle these conditions.)

I am a failure: Imagine a person trying to heal himself or herself with the unconscious thought, "I am a failure." It won't work! They have set themselves to fail at self-healing before they even try. Failing repeatedly with the same healing techniques is a typical pattern that this person would manifest to prove the thought, "I am a failure." Of course this pattern brings up the death urge and their condition truly will get worse fast.

There is something wrong with me: This personal lie is a pretty obvious and sure bet that something wrong will be created in the body. For example, I have known several women with fertility problems that had the "something wrong with me" syndrome. They would run from doctor to doctor trying to get "proof" of infertility. It would drive them nuts if the doctors found nothing wrong. What they were not seeing is that the infertility problem was a result of their thought and, actually, there was nothing wrong at all. I have known women with fertility problems who had given themselves up as hopeless; yet, when they had been Rebirthed and had breathed out that thought, they became pregnant!

I am a disappointment: These people will often set it up to be a disappointment to their parents and mates, bosses and friends, etc. The resulting sadness of all this can make them ill quite easily. They might seek help for the illness but be disappointed in the doctor, the treatment, the outcome or whatever. They may end up thinking that "nothing works".

I shouldn't be here: This personal lie can really be deadly because these persons have quite a death urge and may go around creating near-fatal accidents and illnesses. These people live more often than not on the edge of personal disaster. They may go around bragging to others about how many "near misses" they have had with death. Some of the AIDS patients that I have Rebirthed harbored this thought. (This thought can be changed. However, these persons have to start thinking that they deserve to be alive. It is a drastic shift in energy!) Some of these people have a lot of "out-of-body" experiences and might even be great clairvoyants. However, when these kind of people get really sick, it can be hard for the doctors trying to keep them here on this plane.

I am unwanted: People with this thought pattern are often attracted to people of the opposite sex who are not attracted to them so they can feel "unwanted". The sadness of constant rejection can make them feel devastated and sick, of course. The problem is compounded because often they cannot ask for the support that they need to be healed; they believe other people do not want to help them since they are usually unwanted.

I am evil: This is a core belief, usually brought in from a past life or several past lives. People of this type are very hard on themselves and believe that they deserve severe punishment. They might unconsciously destroy everything good in their lives - businesses, relationships and even their bodies. They cannot ever imagine that they might deserve happiness and success. These people usually need a lot of spiritual help. Some women who were former prostitutes have this thought. Even though they may not be prostitutes in this life, they might tend to manifest attributes of one to make others believe that they are as evil as they believe themselves to be. It is common for these people to create incurable diseases to keep others away, feeling that they deserve no healing whatsoever.

I am stuck: This person may have actually been stuck in the birth canal. Later they get stuck in all kinds of life situations, or stuck with an ongoing weight problem. Their minds may go in vicious circles trying to figure out how to change, but they often get nowhere because they get stuck.

I am nothing: These people have very low self-esteem; they may think that they deserve nothing. Often they manifest anorexia or other diseases that waste away the body. The sad part is that they almost never reach out for help, for they truly believe that nothing or no one exists out there to help them. They may even turn atheistic and deny the love and support of God and the universe. This is a very dangerous negative thought pattern; some of these people really believe that they are nothing and that nothing can help them.

Although all of the negative thought patterns mentioned above sound rather extreme, the truth is that these patterns are more common than most people realize and Rebirthers see them day-in and day-out. For over two decades, I have watched people wrestle with these deep-rooted thoughts and their effects. To Rebirthers, changing these thought patterns is not so grim as it may seem. Rebirthers themselves have gone through their own Rebirthing, discovered their own personal lies and have survived. On the other side of these thoughts is a whole new life!

Often we hear of the death of someone who had been a very happy, healthy and positive person. They may not even have been very old. People may say, "I just cannot understand why one so healthy died, loving life so much." Even people who appear happy and healthy may have deep-rooted negative thought patterns carried from birth or past lives that are silently and secretly running their present lives. Now you might have an insight into the person's early death or it could be past-life karma of course. Rebirthing might prevent early death!

You could be one of the best healers in the world (and if you are, I salute you and hope to meet you someday), but all your work with a client can go down the drain if they go back into their addictions and personal lies. For your work to have more lasting or permanent effect, please consider suggesting Rebirthing to your clients. They will appreciate you all the more, and your healing service will be more valuable in the end. Please consider Rebirthing for yourselves. Your own healing abilities will greatly improve after you discover your own birth and past-life thought patterns. If you are getting good results now, imagine what you might get after eliminating your own personal lies.

A well-trained Rebirther will go after the "personal lies" in the very first session with a client. For a list of LRT sponsored Rebirthers in your area, see the end of this book.

Family Loyalty

You may think that you do not want to copy your parents, especially not their *ailments*. Of course none of us wants to do that! But we feel a very deep loyalty to our parents even if we have not felt close to them. In Rebirthing, we have seen family loyalty take an unconscious form of copying not only parental behavior patterns but also of copying parental illness and death patterns. It is all an unconscious process and an unhealthy form of "loving" that does not make any sense at all. People that are natural conformists manifest these patterns frequently. Rebels, on the other hand, are less likely to manifest them. However, everyone is susceptible to "family loyalty".

When it comes to disease, many people will say that they inherited theirs. They may believe that their disease is genetic and that there is nothing they can do about it. But what if we could acknowledge the fact that we *choose* to go into agreement with our parents and the genes of our parents? What if we could change our genes and that parental agreement *with our minds*? Well, you may think that this is preposterous, but I know of cases where it has been done!

I once went out with a lawyer from Texas whose whole family had Huntington's Chorea. By all odds, he was supposed to have it, too. It is a horrible disease of dementia. He told me about the day that he *chose* not to go into agreement with that disease. It was such a powerful experience for him that he could remember perfectly the day and time of his decision. He could remember everything that was in the room where he was at the time - the color and design of the carpet, curtains and everything. To this day, his family doctors are mystified by his case and can't understand how he beat the odds. He was twelve years old when he made that decision.

Shouldn't this story say something about what we tell our children? If we pass on our negative thoughts to them, they surely will have to struggle to overcome all the potential illness, failure and unhappiness that these thoughts tend to manifest. How do we know when it is too late to change our genes? Is it ever too late? Miracle healings are happening all the time and all over the world. I strongly recommend that you read *Quantum Healing* by Dr. Deepak Chopra if you still have doubts about the power of the mind to change the body.

Many people have already unconsciously programmed their own death to match that of a parent, grandparent or loved one. This then perpetuates the notion that you cannot do anything about inherited diseases. The statistics of such diseases then climb higher and higher and that in turn perpetuates the programming even more. Have you even considered how early we start our conscious and unconscious programming? In my seminars on Physical Immortality, I ask people to write down at what age they think they will die and of what condition. Their answers usually come out quite easily because their decisions were made when they were children! When I ask them why they hold that belief about their death, they often reply that it is because of their first funeral experience, the death of a grandparent or loved one. The conditioning thought was, "I guess I will be like him or her." A person can identify with a parent or grandparent so strongly that they take on that body type - thought process and all.

A person's genetics can change! And I have learned that a person's palm can reveal their genetics. One of my gurus is also a palmist. He reads my palm once every seven years or so because the genetic information changes, according to him. Once I met a man in Russia who had no lines at all on his palm. There was just a little "X" in the middle. I freaked out! I asked him what it meant.

"Total mutation," he said.

He also told me that he had waited all his life to find another person who understood Physical Immortality like I did. (He fell in love with me, but he did not know one word of English and I didn't know Russian!)

Once in a healing seminar that I presented, I had a vision of a new healing process right on the spot: I had two people sit across from each other and record on paper all the symptoms and diseases that their mothers had had, which ones of those they had copied and why they had copied them. Then I had them do the same for their fathers and then for their grandparents. It was a lengthy process which grew so intense that I decided never to do it again unless there was an immediate Rebirthing session afterwards. I found myself personally doing the new process for weeks after that seminar. I processed out all the disease programming that my grandmother had had in her body . Had I not been able to do Rebirthing each step of the way, I am sure I would

have ended up with early, permanent aging. Many
times in my life I had manifested premature aging and
reversed it. (You might want to read my book, *How to
be Chic, Fabulous and Live Forever.*) I considered myself
very lucky to be able to do a follow-up on those students
that experienced my "visionary healing process"! I
have learned now to use these techniques in smaller
doses and only in more advanced classes.

The first step to your mastering this pattern of exces-
sive family loyalty is to recognize your tendency to
copy. If you start getting a disease similar to that of one
of your parents', grandparents' or ancestors', you do
not have to resign yourself to that disease. Resignation
can be deadly. You can rise above the negative thought
patterns. You may need the support of knowledgeable
and advanced healers who know how to transform the
mind and move energy.

The point is: **You can still love your parents without
being loyal to all their patterns***!*

In my case, I was a rebel. My sister was a conformist.
(She actually died at the same age that my father was
when he died.) However, a very strange thing happened to me after she died. I began to switch over to
being a conformist, perhaps to fill the gap somehow for
my mother. It felt very strange and did not work for me
at all. The whole experience threw me into confusion
for a while and I did not know who I really was. I started
to lose my grip. I started to take on my sister's mind, her
disease and what not. I also felt guilty that I was living
and she was not, and I made up ways to suffer for this

guilt. It took me nearly five years to straighten myself out and let those patterns go. It was all an unconscious process and I found it was amazing as I watched it all play out.

Never underestimate the power of the subconscious mind trickery of the ego. Why do you suppose that the Masters strongly recommend that we stay on the spiritual path? We have to be alert, for one thing. And we have to learn the techniques to handle all of the unconscious stuff, for another thing.

I am not a geneticist and I do not want to get in any arguments with geneticists. All I want to point out is this: If someone can materialize his body and demateri-alize his body at will, as I have witnessed my guru Babaji do, then there is a lot about the human mind we don't understand!

If you still think that all of this is crazy, then try reading some of the books written about the ancient teachings of the masters in India. I strongly recom-mend the series by Robert E. Svobada entitled *At the Left Hand of God and the Kundalini*. I can tell you that it is incredible material and I can hardly digest it. What these writings have taught me is that there is something far beyond modern science. There is the Divine Mother - the Eternal One who is Supreme and the Great Healer. If you are stuck in a family disease, start praying to the Divine Mother!

Addiction to Suffering

I had never noticed that I had such an insidious addiction to suffering until recently. That was because, when I compared myself to most people, it seemed that I was doing okay. Yes, I had gone through a lot of devastating experiences, and I had had a lot of unhealthy conditions in my body; but at least I was not in and out of hospitals, etc. I felt quite resilient. I felt pleased that I had not become bitter because of the trials of life. I was not depressed nor moody; in fact most of the time I was happy despite my symptoms. I felt so fortunate that I could travel about freely; even though I was not rich, I had just enough money. Therefore I never counted my symptoms as a form of suffering. I just blamed them on overwork. However, this mistake kept me from facing the area of my mind that I needed to face.

When I got really serious about healing ALL of my symptoms, I had to do an in-depth study of myself to learn why I was not letting them go. Then I discovered that because of my religious upbringing, I thought that I needed to suffer in some way because the Church said suffering is "holy". If I wanted to be "holy" - and I did - then I could never have the perfect life, free of suffering. "If you suffer now, you get to Heaven later," I remembered them saying. (What a brainwashing for torture!) So there I was - always making sure I had some symptom around. I would heal one and then just accept another. That way I could also make sure I was not perfect.

As I grew enlightened and happier and happier, it seemed I should somehow suffer even *more* because of the guilt of being happy. (In Church, somehow you are not supposed to be too happy.) So then it turned out that the happier I grew, the worse my symptoms became...so that I could not stay happy. That was insane!!! I started resenting the Church again - a dangerous attitude, according to Church warnings. If you dare to question the Church, you will surely suffer - and even more later!

Oh, I was able to function all right. I was able to work and even have a fairly good time...but there was always something that kept me from experiencing ecstasy. It seemed to elude me. And that something turned out to be my ego, of course...mainly the part of my ego that was trying to convince me that I had to suffer.

After I recognized this pattern and started to give it up, my mind went into the next phase: A new reason to suffer! Others were suffering. I should be like others if I am to be here and want to be close to them. After all, I could not be the only one around in perfect health! I would be too different. I was already too different. People might think I was a fake. So I had better suffer somewhat in order to be accepted, to be considered "normal". This was the next trick of my ego.

On top of all this nonsense, somehow I had it wired up that if I had symptoms like my father and sister, both of whom had died, I would somehow still be "connected" to them. If I got totally healed, I might want to stay here and then I might not get to go to "Heaven" and be with them again. Furthermore, I felt guilty that I was able to live, and that guilt made more symptoms. All this was unconscious, mind you. It is a wonder I did not land in the hospital. I had to stay on top of it constantly for that not to happen. It was work. Fortunately, I had read *A Course in Miracles* which says, "God's will for us is perfect happiness." This book, which is a correction of religious thought, helped me to straighten out this MESS. I have never given up the full examination of this issue and I am still examining it now.

Then, one day in India, while visiting the great Saint Shastriji, I noticed that he was always in ecstasy. He was never suffering. Besides, he kept shouting to me, "I WANT YOU TO HAVE INTENSE JOY!" Now, try to imagine the effect that had on me. There he was - the living example of what I wanted to be right in front of me. That is what I needed to see, what I needed to hear. And it was REAL. That is why I had gone to India in the first place: I needed to see examples. In one's spiritual life, such experience is called "The Principle of Right Association", i.e., you associate with that which you want to become. You hang out with those who force you to *adapt upward*.

So then, I recommend that you become aware of all the forms of suffering that you might be creating. One can create suffering anywhere - in the body, at work, in a relationship, even on vacation. Become committed to giving up suffering. Talk to Jesus about it, to Babaji, to the Divine Mother. Pray about it. This process should also help you become aware of all that you feel guilty about. (See chapter ahead on guilt and sickness.)

Read *A Course In Miracles* until you unravel false

religious theology. There IS a way out. Keep studying it until you absolutely know that you are innocent and that guilt is not of God.

For meditation, study *The Course in Miracles* lessons:

"God's will for me is perfect happiness."

"I choose the joy of God instead of pain."

"Other people's suffering is not my own."

You may also have to focus forgiveness on the Church and your ministers and teachers who misprogrammed you. Forgive yourself for "buying" it. You knew as a kid that something was really OFF about that, didn't you, really? We try to please our authority figures. If we challenge them as kids, we usually get put down. If you stood up to them as a kid, good for you. If they put you down for it, forgive that, too.

Anger

Anger is very damaging to your etheric substances and organs. It is also damaging to your relationships. When your relationships break down, your body breaks down. *A Course in Miracles* says, "Anger provokes separation, and communication ends separation." *A Course in Miracles* also says, "Anger is never justified."

So what do you do about anger? I have written a lot about this in *Loving Relationships Book II.* However, some of it is worth repeating here: Anger should not be suppressed; that is bad for your body. But if it is expressed, that is bad for others. So you need a way to handle this dilemma. My teacher Babaji gave me the way. He said that what you need to do is change the thought that causes the anger. Are you willing to do that for the sake of your health?

A lot of people might protest this technique, saying that the anger overtakes them too quickly - before they can change the thought. However, this is a discipline that can be learned if one is willing to try. What you do first is notice the feeling of anger coming up. Then you immediately start breathing out the heavy energy and you try to change the thought coming up. It is really not hard, if you put consciousness to it. It helps to have been Rebirthed so that you know how to exhale anger and grow use to observing your thoughts and changing them.

Example: You can actually say:

"I am feeling anger now about................................."

"This is my thought..."

"I am going to run around the block, get Rebirthed, scream in the shower, or whatever."
You change the thought then and there. You do not have to dump the anger on someone else. That is just a bad habit. As you get quicker at this process, and learn to change the thought sooner, the anger will actually dissolve right then if you are willing. Besides, it is probably not really *them* that is making you angry. It is probably someone whom they represent in your past. Furthermore, you might be antagonizing them just to have an excuse to fight. What is your part in provoking this?
I was conducting a marriage consultation once, and the husband told me that he did not have to be the one to ask for forgiveness, because she, his wife started the argument. Therefore it was all her fault. I had to practically go over the whole LRT for him to understand that both were co-creating that moment. He could not express any feelings. He caused her to express double feelings. What he suppressed, she expressed. He needed her to do that so that he could re-create his childhood and feel what was "familiar". She was, of course, just as responsible. We all co-create every moment.
Imagine putting a little baby in a pressure cooker

that was on all the time. Would you do it? Of course not! So why would you do that to your body? You should always be treating your body as kindly as you would a little baby's. I don't even let my body stay in the space of other people's anger. If anyone starts yelling and screaming, I leave. I am too sensitive. Of course I would look at my part of that dilemma, but I can look at my part of that outside the room and protect my body. After all, we do have free will to put our bodies where we want.

I hope that now I am at peace enough that all people around me feel that peace and want to be at peace in my presence. (That does not mean there is no excitement.) People who can maintain high levels of love and excitement and ecstasy without quickly blowing up afterward are getting somewhere. That probably means their subconscious is clear of anger. They can maintain peace in high energy. High energy tends to bring up anything unlike itself. You can tell a lot about people by watching them in high energy situations, and especially afterward. They might go nuts for days afterward. It is absolutely not true that you cannot control your anger. Who IS in control of it? Of course you are. To think that you are not is a cop-out.

Here is what some Gurus say on the subject:

Guru Mai:
    "It is said that if you are a true ascetic, you are completely devoid of anger. If there is any trace of anger in you, you are called a scoundrel, not an ascetic. A great being will go to any extent to remove the fire of

anger. The greatness of a Saddhu Monk is that he can drop something once he realizes he has it."

Dalai Lama:
"We lose control of our mind through hatred and anger. If our minds are dominated by anger, we will lose the best part of human intelligence - wisdom! Anger is one of the most serious problems facing the world today." (Page 12: *A Human Approach to World Peace.* A pamphlet)

Mata Amritanandamayi (The Mother)
"Anger and impatience will always cause problems. Suppose you have a weakness of getting angry easily. Once you become normal again, go and sit in the family shrine room or in solitude and regret and repent your anger. Sincerely pray to your beloved deity or Mother Nature, seeking help to get rid of it. *TRY TO MAKE YOUR OWN MIND AWARE OF THE BAD OUTCOME OF ANGER.* When you are angry at someone, you lose all your mental balance. Your discriminative power completely stops functioning. You say whatever comes into your mind and act accordingly. You may even utter crude words.

By acting and thinking with anger, you lose a lot of good energy. Become aware that these negative feel-ings will only pave the way for your own destruction!" (*Awaken, Children* p. 4-5)

What to do during an ANGER ATTACK

1. *Do not yell at anyone else.*

2. *Lie down and Breathe, pumping out your anger on the exhale.*
(It helps to know the Rebirthing Breath.)

3. *If that does not work, run around the block until calm.*

4. *When you calm down, remind yourself of these two lines from* **A Course in Miracles**:

A. *"You will attack what does not satisfy you to avoid seeing that you created it."*

B. *"Beware of the temptation to perceive yourself as unjustly treated."*

5. *THIS MEANS THAT YOU CREATED THE RESULT AT WHICH YOU ARE ANGRY. YOU SOMEHOW WANTED IT, NEEDED IT OR ARE ADDICTED TO IT. SO TRY TO GET ENLIGHTENED ABOUT THIS FACT AND SEE YOUR PART!*
(What is your payoff? What are you getting out of this that is neurotic?)

6. *Express yourself now sanely.*

A*"I felt angry because..."*

B. *"I see now that I had the thought....................... that attracted this situation."*

C. *"I apologize for this and I want to repent."*

7. *Do the former process recommended by the Mother, Mata Amritanandamayi in a Holy area.*

8. *If you are not completely calm, write down all your feelings of anger and then burn the paper.*

9. *If the above does not work, you need more help. Call a friend who is more enlightened than you at the time to get help "processing."*

10. *Do a truth process such as:* "The reason I do not want to forgive is..................." (Usually seeing your part in the situation dilutes the problem quite a bit if you are telling the truth.)

11. *Remember that forgiveness is the key to happiness and health.*

12. *Remember that behind every grievance, there is a miracle.*

13. *Remember that anger is one of the causes of aging and death.* (It is NOT worth it.)

14. *Follow Catherine Ponders steps to forgiveness*:
A. You forgive them.
B. You forgive yourself.
C. Allow them to forgive you.
D. Give up all desire to punish and get even.
E. Restore good harmony as before the upset.

Guilt and Sickness

Guilt demands punishment - that is, in your ego mind, you believe that that is so. One of the ways we punish ourselves when we feel guilty is to get sick. We attack our bodies then with an illness, pain, or injury which we actually make up.

The *Course in Miracles* says that guilt is not only not of God, it is actually an attack on God! It says that it is a sure sign that your thinking is unnatural. This is all explained in a section called , "The Ego's Use of Guilt." The *Course* also says that if you have guilt, you are walking the carpet of death. (That means that we think we eventually have to die as a form of punishment for our guilt, especially since we think we are such sinners! We therefore kill ourselves with our own thoughts, squeezing the life force right out of ourselves.)

Sometimes, however, you may not even realize you are guilty until you get a symptom. In this way, the symptoms are serving you to make you aware of the guilt. A few years back I developed a lot of tension as a result of having to fire someone. It is the part of my job as a leader that I hate the most. I figured out that the tension was due to the guilt, but I could not seem to shake it. So I discussed it with someone more spiritually advanced at that moment. That teacher gave me some real feedback. He said, "Your problem as a leader is that you don't ever let people fall on their faces." He made it clear to me that some people set it up that way to finally learn their lessons...in effect, they "fire" themselves! I appreciated that teaching from him and I did not let his criticism of me incur more guilt and tensions. I welcome criticism, especially when I need it. So, the moral of the story is: If you cannot get off your guilt, get spiritual help before you destroy your body.

Reading the *Course In Miracles* also helps you get regrounded in your innocence. The *Course in Miracles* says that you can have forgiveness in the "Holy Instant" because God does not make your sins real. ("Sins" means your "case", your "mistakes".) That is because God knows that your "case" is just your ego and that it is not real. This may seem like an advanced concept if you have not read the whole *Course In Miracles*. Another way of saying this is, "Your ego is a nightmare you are temporarily having." You think you are separate (ego); but that is not real. (When your child is having a nightmare, for example, you don't make IT real...nor does God make our nightmares real.) It is important to keep studying the CIM (*Course in Miracles*) until you fully understand this point.

Along with the idea of guilt, one must beware of the danger of carrying "deep dark secrets". This would be like having inside you a festering boil full of guilt that you pretend you do not have and that is not affecting your body! This will keep eating away at you...no doubt about it. You must be willing to tell someone if you have some deep secret you feel guilty about. That was one of the whole ideas of going to a priest. However, confession has in many cases been used to make one feel even more guilty. It might be better to share your dark secret with someone you really trust. Get it off your chest.

An acquaintance of mine was killed in a small plane crash. I had a lot of trouble understanding why he had crashed because he was quite enlightened; I wanted to know what went wrong with his mind to attract that fate. I begged one of my teachers (who is a seer) to tell me. He was reluctant; but after he saw the insomnia I suffered because of that death, he said that this man had a deep dark secret. I later found out that he was in fact, a very secretive person. In the end, this did him in because he never released all his guilt. He tried to hide it.

So, I started teaching my students to confess their deep secrets. One girl finally told the whole group her father was in the Mafia! Her whole life changed after that. She became younger and very powerful in her own right.

Once I did something that I thought was really stupid, and I could not let go of it. One friend knew about it but it still was not enough for me to tell just him. He realized that I needed some kind of "ceremony". So he put me in his car and drove me out in the woods to meet a friend of his, an actual recluse. He told me to go into the shack and confess this thing to his friend, the recluse. Well, I did it. I have no idea who that recluse was or is to this day, but he was very loving. He did not know who I was either, and he did not care. He just heard what I said and loved me and did not bat an eye. He thought it was trivia. I obviously got over the whole thing by confessing, because I cannot even remember what it was about now.

Years later I found myself with a very silly habit that I was really embarrassed about. I could not seem to overcome it for a whole year; and since I was a public figure, I did not want to tell anyone. It was too embarrassing. But then I remembered the friend who had driven me to see the recluse. I went to see him. He was hanging out in a kitchen with another wild friend in San Diego. Now, this guy was the opposite of a recluse. He was rich and all that, and he was "cool". I decided this was the moment and I had to do it; I blurted it out. I was so embarrassed. They looked at me and they both said in unison, "So what?" Then they went right on to something else a lot more interesting! The next day I was cured. The habit disappeared from my life forever.

Find a stranger if there is no one else to talk to. Try it!

Fear and Sickness
My own summary from a year of studying
A Course in Miracles

The *Course In Miracles* says all healing is essentially the release from Fear. It also says there are only two true emotions: Love and Fear. Love is God. That won't make you sick. Fear is Ego. That WILL make you sick.

Fear may seem beyond your control, but it is not. Fear is self-controlled. We ARE responsible for what we think. When we have fear, the *CIM* says, it is a sure sign that we have allowed our minds to miscreate. When we are fearful, we have chosen wrongly. The correction of fear, then, is *our* responsibility. When we ask God to take away our fear, we are implying that it is not our responsibility. We must ask instead for help in the conditions that have brought our fears about. A condition which produces fear, according to the *Course*, is our desire to remain separate from God. Our fear prevents us from letting the Holy Spirit be in charge. If we let the Holy Spirit be in charge, there will be no fear. Fear is, then, a result of our "control number".

The *Course* says that attempting to "master" fear is useless because that gives fear more power. The only way to overcome fear is to master love. Fear comes from thoughts. By choosing loving thoughts you are rejecting fear. In the *Course*, Jesus offers these steps to the release of fear:

1. *Know first that this is fear.*

2. *Fear arises from lack of love.*

3. *The only remedy for lack of love is perfect love.*

4. *Perfect love is the Atonement.*

In the *Course*, the Atonement means allowing the Holy Spirit to correct all your wrong thinking.

Here is a really powerful quotation from the *Course:*

> *"I (Jesus) know it (fear) does not exist; but you do not. You believe in the power of what does not exist."*

What He is saying is that fear does not really exist because fear is the ego, and the ego is separation; the separation does not exist. But we have made the separation appear to be real, and therefore we have made the ego appear to be real. Therefore we have made fear seem real. If we, in fact, think we are separate from God, we are going to have fear.

Anytime we are sick, we are replacing God with the ego. The part of our body that is suffering is where we are storing our ego and pushing out God. That is why the *Course in Miracles* says that "Sickness is idolatry". It actually goes so far as to say that when you are sick, you are trying to kill God.

The body cannot act wrongly unless it is responding to mis-thoughts. It is your thoughts alone that cause you pain and sickness. It is a fundamental error to think that the body creates. The *Course* will tell you this over and over: that if you are sick you are withdrawing from God. You are spiritually deprived. It will tell you over and over that all forms of illness are physical expressions of fear.

There is the fear that causes the sickness and then there is the fear of healing on top of that. The reason healing is a threat is that it would mean that you ARE responsible for your thoughts. In other words, the mind makes the decision to be sick and all illness is mental illness. People often do not want to face this fact. They would rather blame something outside of themselves. It seems easier. However, if you keep doing that, how can you ever heal yourself?

People are often afraid of healing because if they have chosen sickness as a way of life to get attention, they might lose that attention and get really depressed.

People are often very afraid of the miracle healings that they say they want. They may pray for a miracle, but actually they are terrified of miracles. That is because experiencing a miracle would change their whole reality. The thought of accepting a miracle is terrifying to most people. So the *Course* recommends that you understand clearly how to pray for healing. It recommends that you do not pray for a miracle healing of your cancer or arthritis to happen overnight. You have too much fear of that much light, of that much reality shifting that fast. You most likely would not let it happen unless you were in the presence of Jesus Himself or Mary at the Shrine where you would feel completely safe.

In the *Course*, Jesus says to pray for the *removal of the fear of healing* first. After all, the Holy Spirit is not going to *add* to your fear! If you are terrified of miracles, He is not going to scare the hell out of you with one. You have to prepare your mind. You have to be ready for miracles. You have to be over the fear of healing before you will let it happen.

It took me a long, long time to understand these points in the *CIM*. When I finally integrated this information, I was able to adjust the techniques that I explain later in this book. In other words, if you are not giving up a condition, you have to find out why you *fear* giving up that condition. (Don't worry; this will all become more clear to you later on.)

Misery, pain, suffering and death - we are all used to them. We are also addicted to them. (Ego) What we are really afraid of is Life, God and Love. So this makes us hang onto conditions that "bring us down in energy" - to a state that is more familiar than all the energy we would have in a state of absolute pristine and perfect health or in the incredible light-energy of a miracle.

We are so confused that we actually think God kills people. If God is energy, then in that way of thinking, energy kills people. So we are also terrified of energy. And yet the truth is, the energy of God can heal you completely. But you have to get your mind straight first or you will stop the whole process.

The Atonement cures all sickness, Jesus said. The Atonement takes away guilt. Your cure comes from your holiness.

Suppressing fear causes pain. Feel the fear, breathe it out and change the thoughts that cause it. It is the same treatment I gave you for anger. Ask for correction in the *cause* of your fear and your fearful thoughts. The cause is the belief in separation. The only thing you need to correct is your *imagined* separation.

This section you may need to read several times. I wrote it in ten minutes with "Ave Maria" turned up very loud so that I would not be blocked and get my own mind in the way.

The Unconscious Death Urge

One of the *main* causes of sickness and symptoms is what we call the Unconscious Death Urge. This is the ego in its worst form. It includes the following:

The thought,"I am separate from God".

The belief that,"Death is inevitable".

All your programming from society and family about death.

Your family patterns on disease, aging and death.

The invalidation of your personal divinity.

Addictions and bad habits leading to aging and death.

Any anti-life thoughts.

Your secret wish to die because you hate your life.

False religious theology.

Past-life memories of dying, etc., is what we call worst form.

This is like a *conglomerate* in your subconscious mind. It will run you until you take charge of your mind and clear it. This can be done. In every religious tradition there are the Great Immortals who overcame death.

(See later section on Physical Immortality.)

If you constantly affirm, "Death is inevitable," then death is the result you will get. The way to create death is to create aging and sickness so you can die. In the Bible, Jesus actually said: "The power of life and death are in the tongue." That of course means: What you *say* is what you *get* in your body. You are at cause over your body . Your body is like a computer print out; you are the programmer!

Most people believe that death is beyond their control. Some blame it on God. But if you believe that God controls your death, then you are making God a murderer! Others blame "something out there" in the Universe as if "something" is out to get them. If that is the case, it is impossible to walk around in the universe and relax. Your physical body is going to break down with all this tension of wondering when "it" is going to "get you". Besides, if you are trying to live while having the thought that "Death Is Inevitable," it is like trying to drive a car at 90 mph forward with the gears in reverse. It strips the gears. The car breaks down. Your body will break down. Of course, you can also use accidents as a way to kill yourself.

Your physical body is obviously your most valuable possession. However, have you noticed that people take better care of their cars and houses than they do of their own bodies? People allow their bodies to be destroyed, and sometimes easily, without protest.

Actually, it is your *mind* that kills your body. Therefore all death is suicide! The *CIM* says, "Death is a result of a thought called the Ego." People use their egos to kill themselves. If you believe that death is inevitable, then you are in the process of dying right now. You are programming it right now. If you heal one disease and do not change that thought, then you will just make up another one to kill yourself. That is why Leonard Orr, the founder of Rebirthing, said, "All healing is temporary until you heal death." What is the point of learning to heal yourself, then, if you are just going to keep trying to kill yourself?

The minute we forgot who we were and created the fall (separation-ego), death was invented as our own punishment for that "sin". The belief in sin is the self-command for punishment and death. Once you accept the idea that you are separate from God, it is all down-hill after that. Then you will have thoughts like, "I don't have any power. I am weak. I cannot heal myself. I don't deserve life."

Our society is raised in "deathist" mentality. We are hypnotized by the thought that death is inevitable. This belief system is like many belief systems...something we were taught. We think belief systems make us feel safe...even if they are killing us! This is a false sense of safety. Are you willing to change a belief system? When you get outside of belief systems you start experiencing mastery. You go to *direct knowing*. And that is thrilling.

Most people cannot imagine wanting to live forever and giving up their death urge because they are in so much pain. What they do not realize is that the reason they are in pain in the first place is because of their death urge. It is a Catch 22 that one has to figure out.

Your death urge could be operating in many areas of your life. The obvious one is your body. However you could also be "killing off" your relationship, your business, your friendships and what not. You could be losing money in investments because you are killing them off. Never underestimate the power of the ego and the death urge.

Later on in this book I will present more information showing how to use the knowledge of Physical Immortality as a healing force in your body and life. For now, it is important to really see that the death urge is causing disease. It is not the other way around. People think they get sick, age and then die. What they really do is die in their mind and this causes sickness and aging.

One main point of the *Course in Miracles* is that hell is what the ego makes of the present. We create our own hells with our ego and then, after misusing our power and creating hell, we think we deserve to die. In our minds, death becomes the only way out. And according to our egos, we don't think we deserve to live even if we wanted to! Usually we don't want to because we turned our life into hell: pain, misery, suffering and aging. The *Course* spends a long time showing you your "Descent into Hell". To get out of all this, you have to become a Master...but that was the whole point of your life in the first place!

Past Lives and Sickness

I was not aware of the effects of past lives when I was young. I did not even know about the subject! It was certainly not something ever discussed in church (even though I now have found references in the Bible about masters who had lived "before" as someone else). And this topic was certainly not something discussed in medicine when I studied nursing.

When I finally made it to California in the 70's, I was, of course, compelled to read books such as Edgar Cayce's which really opened me up to past-life ideas. And after Rebirthing started, I had to look at the subject more closely. One day I had a client who began remembering being in a war in Ireland. She suddenly began speaking perfect Irish during the session. She certainly was not Irish in this life...that was obvious. Later I asked her if she had ever been to Ireland and she said, "No". I asked her if she had ever studied the Irish language and she said, "No". I asked her if she remembered speaking to me in long paragraphs in Irish without hesitation. She was able to remember the scenes, but only vaguely the speaking.

Also, some time after that, I began to have more and more past-life memories in my own Rebirthing sessions. I would see scenes that were clearly from other eras, and nothing that I had ever glimpsed in any movie, either. The styles of furniture and architecture were very different from anything I had known in my current life. The main thing that always amazed me was that I would have such strong emotions when having those memories. They were so spontaneous and real to me that I knew that I could not be making that up. It was too strong. Why would I want to make that up anyway? I started paying attention.

Then I went to India for the first time. It was after that visit that I began to have past-life memories frequently. It was as if my guru, Babaji, were deliberately pushing them up into my mind to be cleared. There was no way I could avoid this clearing, whether I liked it or not. And it has been going on for years and years now. Recently the much more difficult ones have come up.

Now I can relate to many stories told by clients with illnesses they couldn't seem to heal until they came to us for Rebirthing. Quite frankly, I can say that Rebirthing, with a past-life regression, did the trick. We are very happy that this kind of healing is now being adequately and professionally researched. I would definitely refer everyone to the book, *Other Lives, Other Selves* by Dr. Roger Woolger. I called him personally immediately after reading it. This book is a must for all Rebirthers and Healers. I also recommend it to all clients. It is hard to put down. I think it must have made a huge impact on the field of psychology by now. In the first chapter, Dr. Woolger acknowledges that he was a skeptic who encountered his past lives only when he started Rebirthing. The professional studies he has done are truly awesome.

On page 100, Dr. Woolger states:

"The body and its various aches, pains and dysfunctions is a living psychic history when read correctly. Even though the physical ailment may have very specific origins in a person's current life, I have found more and more that there are certain layers to every major syndrome of physical illness, accident, or weakness. The existence of a past life level of physical problems has been confirmed over and over again in the cases I have seen."

On page 101:

"A woman in her early forties relived an unfulfilled life as a woman in the pioneer days which ended tragically when a horse and trap overturned; she broke her back and died when she was twenty-seven in that life. In this life, at age twenty-seven, she was in the hospital with a very serious kidney infection which they could not properly diagnose and she nearly died ...the pain was absolutely terrible and was in the same place where she had broken her back in the other life."

On page 143, he describes his work with PHOBIAS:

"Although many phobias do, indeed, arise in this life, it seems to be the case that almost everyone has some particular deep fear that will not be thus explained. Whether it be fear of spiders, wild animals, fire, water, heights, crowds, knives, dark places, and so on. I have consistently found that behind that fear lies a specific and detailed story of a past-life trauma. In sessions, people remember deaths from poisonous insects, from spiders, snakes, sharks and more. Many who fear heights recall deaths from being thrown off cliffs, falling from planes in recent wars, etc. "

"Increasingly," he says (p. 171), "in practicing psychotherapy from a past-life perspective, I am convinced that the likelihood of cure depends on whether or not I am able to guide my client to the crucial or key story from his or her past lives. My experience indicates that if we can reach such a story in the early session, cure will be correspondingly swift."

This book also contains stories about how gynecological problems related to past lives of sexual abuse and rape. There are many detailed accounts about how these ancient traumas relate to present-day frigidity and lack of orgasm in women.

Woolger, Dr. Roger J., Ph.D., *OTHER LIVES, OTHER SELVES*. Bantam Books. 1988

Part III

Framework for Healing

Your Relationship With Your Symptoms

When you develop symptoms or a disease, there are a number of different ways you might react to the situation:

You might deny this is going on at all.
You might acknowledge it, but avoid it.
You might be angry at the situation.
You might even fight it and get in a battle in your mind.
You might resist it.
You might hate yourself for it.
You might continually complain about it.
You might continually worry about it.
You might even get very obsessed with it.
You might get really depressed about it.
You might overdose with food, liquor or drugs to
suppress it.
You might get terrified of it.
You might mistakenly think it has more power than you.

It is extremely tempting to take one of these approaches, especially if the symptoms are sticking around. The trouble is that "What you resist persists," so these approaches only fortify the symptoms. Remember the metaphysical principle that "What you think about expands!" So the more you dwell on it in a negative way, the worse it will get. True, it IS hard not to dwell on it negatively, especially when it is painful. But it will get even more painful when you dwell on it.

Denying it is not good either. You need to learn from it
and take the necessary action to change.

So then, you really have to get a hold of your mind.
The *Course In Miracles* says that "The Physician is the
mind of the patient himself." This means that you are
your own doctor: You created the symptom and you
can uncreate it. But you must start by giving up the
above tempting tendencies and you must develop a
loving relationship with your symptom or disease.
How to do that? Ah, yes, that is the trick!

First, acknowledge it as a blessing...in that it is there to
show you that your mind is *off*. It is there to teach you
something very important. It is there to teach you that
your mind needs correction. It is there to get your
attention.

Second, ask the symptom, "What are you trying to tell
me?" Or have a friend ask you the question, "If your
symptom could talk, what would it say to you?"
(The answer is within. It is not acceptable to say, "I
don't know." You *do* know. The answer is within. Your
partner or friend should not accept that answer. They
must then say to you, "If you did know, what would it
be?" ("I don't know" comes from not looking.) For
exact information on the cause of this condition, do
the Truth Process in this book. This is a very, very
important step in self-analysis. If you want *Permanent
Healing* you have to know the *Cause*.

Third, try the techniques in this book. If the symptom
or disease does not shift after self-analysis, the Truth

Process and Rebirthing, for example, then you need a lot more understanding of the framework in this book and with the techniques given later in this book. You should go to a Rebirther, for example, and find out why you do not want to be healed.

Fourth, remember that the sickness is the "cure in process". This means that you take the attitude of experiencing your condition as a purging of a negative thought or construct, rather than as something stuck. Taking this attitude is very important - the basis for your healing. You have to train yourself to remember this: Your body is trying to "spit out" the effects of the negative thoughts which caused it. Your body is attempting to cure itself when you have symptoms. You need to mentally cooperate with this healing process. If you fight it, ignore it, or react in one or more of the negative ways mentioned at the beginning of this chapter, you will only add negative mental mass.

Attitude and Frame of Mind

In my opinion, the hardest part of being sick (besides feeling terrible, of course) is the worry that the condition will never end. So often one is tempted to think, "What if I *never* get over this???" This fear could then escalate to the point that you actually start thinking you will definitely never get over this. At that point it may even start feeling like your body is controlling you instead of you controlling it.

When you have overwhelming fear, you forget that you are controlling your body with your mind and you start thinking that your body or disease is controlling you - that it is more powerful than you. Then the situation gets even worse because you feel helpless. You are losing it now and you must take drastic action to realize that *you* are in charge. Your body is never at cause. You are. Your mind is. If you don't correct your mind at this point, you could become paralyzed with fear to the point that the body's automatic healing system would literally shut down. Or you could end up crystallizing the symptom into something very solid. Therefore, it is really important to get through this danger by having the thought: "THIS WILL PASS...."

A person may go from doctor to doctor or from healer to healer with none of them able to help - because part of the person's mind is trying to prove that the condition cannot be healed. That way the person can continue to hate God for his or her "plight" and remain angry rather than changing that all-important attitude. Of course people who "need" their anger rarely admit it. It is their little "secret". Or, they could be in total denial of their war against God. If one were healed and remained healed, and felt fantastic, and everything was working, what would there be to get angry at? Some people just do not want to give up their "right" to blame.

If you are creating the sickness or symptoms because you want attention, then you may not want to be healed either, because you would then lose all the attention. This is another trap! If you are creating the sickness or symptom as a way of suffering because you believe that you *must* suffer, then you might also set it up not to be healed. If you are creating the sickness or symptoms as a way of punishing yourself for something, you will probably set it up not to be healed because you still think you need more punishment.

When you finally see no more value in the pain and suffering and self-punishment, you will spontaneously heal yourself or finally manifest the right doctor or healer to help you do the trick. "The outcome is what the patient decides." It will become spontaneously obvious what you need to do or where you need to go or whom you need to be with to end your ailment. "God is ready when you are." You will probably wonder why it took you so long to recognize the obvious!

Someone said, "You will be sick until you are sick of being sick." Or, you will get off it when you are *ready* to get off it. One day you decide this attention you enjoy from the illness is not worth it. Or you decide you have had enough of an excuse for a break. Or you decide you no longer have any more fear of being in your full power. Or you finally forgive. Or whatever.

Many times students who have already taken my spiritual healing class will come to me and complain about some ailment they have had for a long time. I ask them "Well, what did you get when you did the Ultimate Truth Process?" Then they confess to me that they did not do it!!

I ask "Why not?" Oh!...they *forgot*, they say.

I was always so surprised at this answer at first. But now I understand how tricky the ego is. It will distract you from what works. You have to train yourself to do the Truth Process as soon as you get the symptoms so that they won't escalate. Of course, if you like to suffer or punish yourself, you won't do the Process even if you do remember. Sometimes people "forget" because of a deep unconscious fear of going against the Church that told them they must suffer. That distorts their thinking. In that case, the person needs to be helped by someone like me or someone else who is no longer trapped in that dogma.

The truth process is on page 140.

Finding the Solution

IMPORTANT POINTS:

1. The part of your mind that is *real*, of the Holy Spirit's Mind, totally alive and perfect, is *always* there, and is always stronger than any mistaken thought of your ego. Your ego miscreated the negative condition.

Say, "I am stronger than this............................" or, "The God in me is stronger than............................"

2. Remember again that anything you have created, you can uncreate. It is *actually less work* to heal yourself than to make yourself sick. It takes a lot of effort and struggle to hang on to a lot of negative thinking in order to make yourself sick. Your natural state is health. You had to really work at going against your natural state to have created this condition.

3. Anything on its way up is on its way *out*. That is another way of saying that your symptom is the cure in process. At least it is no longer suppressed!

4. You may need to get a Rebirther sooner than you think - one who knows how to "process" or clean your resistance to healing. The Rebirther should be able to help you get to the cause of the condition, help you breathe it out, and help you process yourself if the healing is not working because you are blocking it.

5. The **WILL TO LIVE** is the most important factor in your healing. If your life urge is strong enough, you definitely can overcome. If you get stuck in the fear, "I might die," you will weaken greatly and inhibit the natural healing abilities of the body. Recently I read an article about a man who had severe metastasis of cancer. He reversed it all and came out clean, much to the shock of doctors who could hardly accept his healing. The one thing I remember about the article is that he said he *never* entertained the thought that he was going to die. Somehow he was able to have absolute certainty - and it worked.

On the plane the other day I read about the longest living AIDS patient who has beat all odds. What I remember about that article is that he used that very same thinking. He decided, and told his mate, that he was not going to die from it. Doctors keep researching this guy to see why he has beaten all odds. But in the research they forget to study that very point! They studied his diet, his habits, his relationships, his living style...everything. The conclusion: Maybe he is still alive because he meditates. They never mentioned his absolute decision to live. I read about that in a different section of the article in which he was talking about himself.

6. Remember: **FAITH IS EVERYTHING!** When your faith is weak and the temptation to think that you won't make it takes over...that is exactly when you need to pray more, get Rebirthed, and get support.

Spiritual Background
The Course in Miracles Review

The *Course in Miracles* is a correction of religion. It is very important to understand how false religious theology is ruining and running our lives. It is very important to understand how it is affecting our minds, our bodies, and our health. Naturally much of what we learned in church was wonderful, however, there were teachings that were intolerably confusing. Until those points are cleared up, it is hard to figure out *Permanent Healing*.

For example, the Church has taught that we are separate from God. This mistaken theology leads us to believe that we must die to be with God; therefore we, of course, get sick and age. We think we are bad for being here because we "left" God to get here. Therefore we are sinners of the worst kind. If we believe this premise, we will have tremendous guilt - and guilt demands punishment. One of the main ways we punish our-selves is by damaging our bodies, getting sick, aging and finally choosing death as the final punishment. The *Course* calls this our descent into hell while here on earth.

The Church has taught us that heaven is somewhere else and is our goal. Therefore, we cannot really wait to leave here and, as a result, we are not fully here. The worst part is that by making statements such as "the Lord took him away" when someone dies, the Church has taught that God kills people. This insanity makes us fear and hate God for taking away our loved ones and for making us feel that God does not permit us to live as long as we would like. The Church has implied that we should not have too much fun or joy. We are supposed to suffer, so we become addicted to having disease.

Therefore, the joy of having *Permanent Healing* is something we think we do not deserve. Confusion after confusion reigns. These confusions leave us tied up in knots. We supposedly are not even allowed to question the Church or we might go to hell. How then can one get anything straight? This is exactly why we need the *Course in Miracles* - to straighten things out.

The *CIM* is not a religion nor a path. It is a correction. When you read it, you will know that it came from Jesus and there is only one appropriate response: gratitude to Him. The reason it is Christian in tone is that Christianity must be corrected first, since it is such a major influence on the planet. There is no body of knowledge that does not need to be corrected and upgraded. However, many religions are threatened by the ideas in the *Course*, because it challenges what is false. Some do not want to change even though they profess that they do not like the horrors afflicting society and that something must be done. Before anyone criticizes the *Course*, I should think they need to read it all the way through. This is common sense. If adverse critics would read it all the way through before criticizing it, I think they would change their tune.

The *Course* explains that everything we know is wrong; so we have to start over. (Our results should show us that.) Everything is wrong because we are interpreting everything through the ego. The ego is a false self that we made up to compete with God. It is based on the erroneous thought: "I am separate from God." Once we believed that, we went into weakness, helplessness, fear, anxiety, suffering, anger, misery, sickness, aging and death.

In the ego's interpretation, this separation is real and it actually happened. Therefore, God is out to destroy us for this. We therefore try to bargain with God, saying, "You don't have to go to the trouble of punishing me; I will punish myself." The idea of sacrifice was then formed: "I will suffer and deprive myself to prove I am good, so you won't be angry, God." In the ego's thought system, we get the insane notion that sacrifice is salvation, that God's will for us is perfect misery, and that we do not deserve to be happy. Furthermore, we think that the more we suffer now, the better off we will be later on (such as in Heaven).

THE EGO'S VERSION IS THAT WE MUST PERISH.
(I acknowledge the great teacher Ken Wapnick, one of the leading experts on the *CIM*, for helping me to understand the *CIM*.)

The ego's interpretation of the Crucifixion is that only one of God's sons (Jesus) had to suffer for all of us to be freed. However, this interpretation has laid more guilt on our heads; i.e., how does it make you feel if someone who is totally pure has to die for you? This interpretation, Ken explained, does not make us feel free of guilt at all; yet salvation is supposed to free us from guilt. Obviously, we do not really understand the Crucifixion. This is again why we need the *Course in Miracles*. It explains that the Crucifixion was an extreme teaching device. It shows that no perception of oneself as a victim is justified. It explains that Jesus did not defend himself, nor did He even believe that He was attacked. He saw only threatened people who did not think they deserved the love of God.

In the *Course,* Jesus is saying that the truth is that there is no sin because there is no separation. The truth is that it is impossible for us to separate from God. Therefore we are innocent. All sins are forgiven because they never really occurred. Therefore there is no need for sacrifice. Since you are innocent, you do not need to suffer; and since that is true, you can also give yourself perfect health now!

Personally, it has taken me a long time to digest the *Course* because I was addicted to the dogma of the Church for so many lifetimes. I, like most people, brought to this life certain core beliefs that seemed impossible to change - such as "we are sinners". It seemed that if I should give up the thought that I am a sinner, then I would *really* be a sinner. Or if I dared think we are innocent, then I *really* would be guilty. This is the *trap* of the ego. What helped me most was to remember this: If there is a lie at the center of a thought system, the whole system is deceptive. Since the "lie" at the center of my religion was that one is separate from God, then I had to admit that the whole religion is off. Even after I understood that, I was still afraid because the Church had an extra built-in control number: If I question that, or tried to leave, I would surely go to hell and die.

But then one day I realized all that this was really ridiculous because, on the one hand, they were using the threat of death to control me, and on the other hand they were promoting death as something to look forward to for final peace! This double-bind was not resolvable and therefore I knew it had to be off. I resented being put into this trap my whole life. I regretted buying into it. Through prayer and help from my teachers, I have been able to unravel this conflict to the point that things make more sense. I know now that many of the illnesses that I have manifested and mentioned in this book, were a direct result of this religious brainwashing and confusion. (Some people are now calling it religious abuse.)

I do not want to be on a campaign to attack religion. I have tried to forgive all false religious theology. What I want is to be able to understand what is false and what is real - and Jesus is telling us NOW. He says that the Holy Spirit was placed in our minds as a solution to our imagined separation. To Jesus, our identity is Spirit. Therefore we are love, joy, happiness, bliss, peace and perfect health. There is even the possibility of Immortality if one follows His words and practices spiritual laws. He even said this in the Bible: "If you follow me, you will never see the grave." Few could do it; however some did and became Immortal masters who ascended (dematerialized).

Often when Immortals try to explain that giving up the death urge is the key to having perfect health and that Physical Immortality is a real possibility, others cannot accept such information because their minds are in the other framework (ego). So it would be like talking to a wall or speaking in a foreign language. In order to understand the idea of *Permanent Healing*, one would have to have one's mind in the opposite framework. One literally must know the difference between the ego's thought system and the Holy Spirit's thought system. (And here we are not talking about Freud's definition of the ego.) People in the ego's thought system will think that death is inevitable - and it will be. They will think death is the will of God.

I have chosen only two paragraphs to quote from the *Course.* If you read them carefully, I think you will be stunned. However all the rest of the *Course* is as astounding. Imagine your awe if you should read the whole *Course*!

The problem is that the ego tries to keep us from learning that which would heal us. So there could be tremendous resistance even to buying the *Course.* There could be more resistance to reading it. The books say that this *Course* is required if you want to make it....Only the time you take is voluntary. Meaning: You can get it in the next five months, the next five years or the next five lifetimes. But, why wait? Why not now?

You could read the following and substitute the word *sickness.* All sickness and symptoms are part of the death urge and ego. Sickness and death are correlative.

"Death is not your Father's will nor yours. The

death penalty is the ego's ultimate goal, for it truly
believes that you are a criminal deserving death. The
death penalty never leaves the ego's mind, for that is
what it always reserves for you in the end. It will
torment you while you live, but its hatred is not
satisfied until you die. As long as you feel guilty,
you are listening to the voice of the ego, which tells
you that you have been treacherous to God and therefore deserve death."

TRY TO STAY WITH THIS...READ IT AS MANY
TIMES AS YOU NEED TO. IT COULD BE THE KEY TO
YOUR HEALING AND HEALTH.

"You will think that death comes from God and not
from the ego, because by confusing yourself with the
ego, you think you want death. When you are tempted
by the desire for death, remember that I DID NOT DIE.
(Jesus speaking) Would I have overcome death for
myself alone? And would eternal life be given to one of
the Father's sons, unless He had also given it to you?
"When you learn to make ME manifest, you will
never see death. God did not make death. But if you use
the world for what is *not* its purpose, you will not escape
the laws of disease, violence and death. "FORGET NOT
THAT THE HEALING OF GOD'S SONS (All SOULS)
IS ALL THE WORLD IS FOR."

"NO ONE CAN DIE UNLESS HE CHOOSES DEATH."
What seems to be the fear of death is really its attrac-
tion.

When you make sin real, you are requesting death. To the ego, sin means death, so atonement is achieved through murder!

"DEATH IS THE RESULT OF THE THOUGHT WE CALL THE EGO, JUST AS SURELY AS LIFE IS THE RESULT OF THE THOUGHT WE CALL GOD."

"Death is an attempt to resolve conflict by not deciding at all. Like any other solution the ego attempts, it will not work. To the ego , the goal is death. The ego is insane."

The *Course* says Hell is what the ego makes of the *present*. The way out of our own hell is to accept The Atonement for ourselves. That means inviting in the Holy Spirit and accepting the correction of all our wrong thinking. It means not giving support or agreement to anyone else's illusions of sickness and death. It means having the right perception of the body.

"When the body becomes an empty space, without any purpose other than the one the Holy Spirit gives it, it can become a sign of life, a promise of redemption, a breath of immortality to those grown sick of breathing in the fetid scent of death. The Will of God, who created neither sin nor death, wills that you not be bound by them."

Jesus goes on to say in the *Course*, that nothing is accomplished through death. Everything is accomplished through life, and life is of the mind and in the mind. He says that if we share the same mind, we can overcome death, because He did.

Physical Immortality
(Summarized from Chapter Six of
Rebirthing in the New Age)

If you have the ability to destroy your body (which takes a whole lot of effort), you can just as well preserve it, which is a great deal easier. However, if you believe that death is inevitable and that you are separate from God, then you are in the process of dying right now.

" Oh," you might say, "a hundred years of this is all I can take." This statement springs from a deep-rooted belief in suffering and limitation. You have not yet experienced the fullness of health, joy, wisdom, peace and love. You are given the means by which to have these substantive qualities of life itself; and once you have them, why leave?

The corollary of death is sickness. By the way, *A Course in Miracles* says that sickness is idolatry!

Some people say, "Well, I am willing to live forever if it does not get too bad." That is a cop-out because it only gets too bad if one has not given up loyalty to death. In other words, the reason one has pain, suffering, misery and a bad time is precisely because of hanging on to the death urge.

People think that you age, you get sick and then you die. The truth is that "You die in your mind, you get sick, and then you age." You create symptoms in your body that make it socially acceptable to leave it.

Your beliefs control your physical body. If you think you are going to die, you will. However, death is *optional*. And there also is an alternative to aging! The key to that is to stop affirming that "Death is inevitable". This will definitely improve your health.

   Choosing life is what strengthens your body the most. That means choosing life so fully that you love it so much you want to live forever. *That kind of passion is what works.* Physical Immortality can be defined as *endless existence*, specifically the endless existence of your physical body in perpetual health and youthfulness. The body may look different...we have to learn about that. It would be a "Diamond Body". (See "The Last Initiation" p.118)

   We are not talking about living in an old body for hundreds of years; we are talking about learning to rejuvenate the body and reverse the aging process. Your body does have the ability to produce new cells. (You have already seen this yourself many times...for example, when you repair a cut.) Your body is a constantly flowing stream of life. It has a built-in regeneration battery. If you are using your mind correctly, you are in charge of how you flow your stream of life.

   Of course if you are tempted by the idea that you are not one with God...and therefore cannot determine the consequences of your own actions...and are not in charge of your own body, then it is all over. Once you invalidate your divinity in this manner and think you are a sinner, then you will go into helplessness and think, "I cannot heal myself," or "I am weak," or "God is going to destroy me since I am so bad."

Spiritual masters do not think like that at all. They constantly remember who they are. That is the difference. Some of them can rapidly age their bodies at will; and some can even transform them into male or female, a child or an elderly person at will. Babaji is an example of such a master. (Read *Autobiography of a Yogi*.) It should be our purpose for all of us to become spiritual masters.

God is not only love, but God is also LIFE. Life without beginning or end. God is not the author of anything that is not Himself. In the Book of Ezekiel we are told that He wills NOT the death of any, but that all should turn to Him and LIVE.

The body is the temple of the Living God. But remember this: It is possible to weaken the soul's hold on the body with the thought that death is inevitable or with the thought that disease is stronger than the power of God. *Don't ever allow yourself to think that any disease is stronger than the power of God!* This is a departure from Divine Mind.

The Bible presents death as the last enemy to be destroyed.

REVELATIONS 21:4
"And God shall wipe away all tears and there shall be no more death..."

AFFIRMATIONS:

I am alive now, therefore my life urges are stronger than my death urges. As long as I continue strengthening my life urges and weakening my death urges, I will go on living in health and youthfulness.

Life is eternal and I am life. My mind, as the thinking quality of life itself, is eternal. My physical body is also eternal. Therefore my living flesh has a natural tendency to live forever in perfect health and youthfulness.

My physical body is a safe and pleasurable place for me to be. The entire universe exists for the purpose of supporting my physical body and for providing a pleasurable place for me to express myself.

All the cells of my body are daily bathed in the perfection of my divine being.

The more I am good to myself, the more I enrich my own aliveness.

The Last Initiation
(This part was given to me in India - from *Being,
Evolution and Immortality* by H. Chaudhuri)

"Finally, the concept of immortality implies a
harmonization of the entire personality and a transformation of the physical organism as an effective
channel of expression of higher values. This may be
called material immortality."

"There are some mystics and spiritual seekers who
strengthen and purify their bodies just enough to be
able to experience the thrilling touch of the Divine.
They use the body as a ladder - climbing towards a
pure spiritual level. On attaining that level, the body is
felt as a burden, as a prison house, as a string of chains
that holds one in bondage. Dissociation from this "last
burden" of the body is considered a *sine qua non* for
total liberation. Continued association with the body
is believed to be the result of the residual trace of
ignorance."

*"The above view is based upon a subtle misconception about
the purpose of life and the significance of the body."*

"The body is not only a ladder that leads to the
realm of immortality of the soul, but also an excellent instrument for expressing the glory of physical
immortality in life and society. It is capable of being
thoroughly penetrated by the Light of the Spirit. It is
capable of being transformed into what has been called
the "Diamond Body". As a result of such transformation,

the body does not appear any more to be a burden upon the liberated self. It shines as the Spirit made Flesh. It functions as a very effective instrument for creative action and realization of higher values in the world. It is purged of all inner tension and conflict. It is liberated from the anxiety of repressed wishes. It is also liberated from the dangerous grip of the death impulse born of self-repression. Mystics who look upon the body as a burden suffer from the anxiety of self-repression and the allurement of the death wish."

"Material immortality means decisive victory over both of these demons. It conquers the latent death instinct in man, and fortifies the Will to Live as long as is necessary, as a channel of expression of the Divine. It also liquidates all forms of self-suppression and self-torture and self-mutilation. As a result, the total being of an individual becomes strong and steady, whole and healthy. There is a free flow of psychic energy. It is increasingly channeled into ways of meaningful self-expression. Under the guidance of the indwelling Light of the Eternal, it produces increasing manifestation of the Spirit in Matter."

Happiness = Health

Many people think or say, "I won't be happy until I am healthy." This is understandable; yet the truth is, you will be healthy when you are happy! If you read Dr. Deepak Chopra's books, especially *Quantum Healing*, this will become very clear to you; he even explains it scientifically. He also makes it clear that unhappiness is due to loss of contact with the Source. That means that you are forgetting that you are one with God.

Mother Theresa says that most people are spiritually deprived and that this is the whole problem with the world. This is very important; yet when people are told to become spiritual in order to be happy, they often rebel. They are likely to think that that means they must go back to something like the church or some kind of dogma. They usually do not want to do so because they rarely have seen it work for their parents and/or they have been very disappointed in religion themselves. This is a tragedy.

Becoming more spiritual is really finding the deeper *Self* which is *Real* - that part that possesses absolute wisdom and self-knowledge. Dr. Chopra says that in India, finding the "knower" is considered life's greatest adventure. Well, that is exactly why I love to go to India each year! I cherish having the opportunity to be with the great saints who are bursting with joy. In one's spiritual life, this is called the "principle of right association" - placing oneself with the highest beings possible so that one is forced to adapt UPWARD!

This past year when I went to visit the great saint, Shastriji, Babaji's High Priest, this is what he said to me as I approached him and his family: "I WANT YOU TO HAVE INTENSE JOY!" That made such a deep impression on me! (Did you know that the mother of our great American comedian, Robin Williams, told him when he was a child that the purpose of life was to have intense joy?? Imagine the blessing of having a parent telling you that at your early age! Parents, take note!)

"*Happiness* derives from the verb 'to happen'. Happiness is to be found simply from observing what happens. If you cannot be happy at the prospect of lunch, you are not likely to find happiness anywhere. What happens is happiness."
(Robert Johnson. *TRANSFORMATION: Understanding the Three Levels of Masculine Consciousness*)

The idea, of course, is to be happy no matter what is going on around you *and* to know how to be happy without your happiness being dependent on material things. You must remember also that all misery is self-inflicted, and that blaming the world for your unhappy situations will never work. All this has to do with handling your mind. Your mind-body system has to be connected with pure consciousness. (In Transcendental Meditation, it is called the "unified field," which is the Source of all energy fields and fundamental particles.) When we are aware of our connection to that, then, as Dr. Chopra says, all existence is experienced once again as bliss.

"Bliss," Maharishi, the founder of Transcendental Meditation, says, "is ultimately the most powerful agent of physiology." Maharishi says that any attempt to treat disease or any form of suffering on the physical level is too superficial. Bliss *is* the fundamental nature of the Self. The method that Maharishi and Deepak Chopra recommend for experiencing the state of bliss is to settle down the mind through Transcendental Meditation.

In my book *PURE JOY*, I have listed many other methods of spiritual purification that help you return to that state of bliss. All this does not mean that you should not try to arrange your life so that you are happy about your surroundings, your job, your relationships and your situations. Of course all that is important, but not anywhere near so important as the state of your mind. You may be in a job that is not right for you and/or a relationship that is not right for you. That is definitely not a good idea. I know many people who are staying in dead or destructive relationships because they are afraid to leave. Staying in a relationship you do not want to be in just because you are afraid to leave, is *not* a good reason to be there. And, is it even ethical?? Staying in a job that makes you unhappy does not make any sense either. If you do not like the way things are in your life, change them! You may have to leave your job, your marriage, your area, or whatever.

WARNING: It may be just your attitude, however; and if you change all these external things and do not change your attitude, the same thing could come up elsewhere. First try loving where you are, whom you are with and what you are doing, and see what happens.

A lot of people are unhappy because they have no idea why they are here nor the purpose of their life. Nothing really "hangs together" for them. There is a lot one could say on this subject...but let's get clear on one thing: The purpose of life is not just to get married, have children and then die. The purpose of life is to recognize the Supreme, according to my teacher Shastriji. (That is entirely another ball of wax.) This means of course, that you really need to think about your priorities. Are you, for example, on the spiritual path of becoming all that you can be?

The formula for happiness from my guru Babaji, is this: LOVE, TRUTH, SIMPLICITY AND SERVICE TO MANKIND. (He also recommended to us the Mantra Om Namaha Shivai for purity.) Do you understand that all work is worship and should be dedicated to God daily? This changes everything, by the way. Think about these things.

"Readiness and willingness to do any work at any time in any circumstance is the hallmark of spirituality. Spiritual people do it with love and sincerity, without expecting anything. That is why there is always a charm and beauty in whatever spiritual people do. They love to do the work, because the work itself gives them infinite happiness. When we keep worrying about the result, the work loses its beauty."

"To derive the full benefit of any action, whatever it may be, love for that particular action is absolutely necessary."
Mata Amritanandamayi, *Awaken Children* (p.260)

This is all great, you might say, but you feel really really depressed...and so you cannot relate to any of this. What about that? Depression can be understood like any other symptom and treated spiritually. You need to find the cause of the depression, and for that you can actually use the same truth process given in this book. The *Course in Miracles* goes so far as to say that all depression (like sickness) is an *idol* that is made up as a substitute for God!

We have found in Rebirthing that the main cause of depression is the "unconscious death urge". (This, as I mentioned earlier, is a "consciousness factor" which includes your programming on death, the thought that death is inevitable, your secret wish to die because you hate your life, past-life memories of dying, the thought "I am separate from God" and other anti-life thoughts.) All of that can surely make a person depressed!

My very first client when I became a Rebirther was a real test for me. She came to me very depressed, telling me she wanted to kill herself. She was very suicidal and she told me she did not want me to try to talk her out of that. She went on and on and on about why she wanted to die. I listened, but then I realized, of course, that the part of her that wanted to live had come to me for Rebirthing. If she truly had wanted to die, she would never have come at all! So I focused on that part of her mind. I honored her wish not to push her to live.

I just asked her to lie down and breathe and I asked her to simply postpone her suicide five days until her next Rebirthing. I checked on her every day. I kept doing this each session until suddenly, after about 8 sessions, she wanted to live. She had breathed out enough death urge in the sessions that she felt different. She later became a dancer! Imagine! Now she is happily married also.

Even if you are a person reading this book who has what has been called a "fatal illness" and you have a "bad prognosis", let me repeat again what Leonard Orr, the founder of Rebirthing said; "As long as you have one breath left, there is still a chance." And he also reminded us that Jesus took it even further and brought people back *after* they had died. For more information on these kinds of cases read *"The Romeo Error".* So NEVER GIVE UP!!

"WITH GOD, ALL THINGS ARE POSSIBLE."
(Matthew 19:26)

You might say, "Right, okay, I have now decided that I do not want to let a boring job, boring life, or boring relationship ruin my body...but how can I guarantee I can get out of these dreary messes?"

Well, what about the *boring mind* aspect that goes before these results? Here is a very interesting statement, again by Leonard Orr:

"Most people fear eternal life more than they do physical death; but what they really fear is not eternal life of their bodies, but the eternal life of their boring minds! The essential characteristic of a boring person is the morbidity of the deathist mentality."

"CONQUERING DEATH IS THE BASIC INTELLIGENCE TEST OF SPIRITUAL ENLIGHTENMENT."

Remember: Deathist mentality is unhealthy for human beings.

Influence of Relationships

A relationship can heal you or damage you more... depending on how you play the game of relationships.

You may want your mate to agree with you on everything and "back you up" no matter what. Or, you as a mate may think that that is what you are required to do as a mate...agree with him or her and back them up no matter what. This could look like a healed relationship....But what if it is just collusion and codependency that you are creating? If so, watch out later. In other words, what if your mate agrees with you just to "make you happy", and what if you were into your ego or "case" at the time? He would then be supporting your case, supporting your ego, supporting that which will eventually make you sick and destroy you! Now that you have someone in agreement with your "case", how is that going to help you and heal you? It's not! You are merely reinforcing what you are supposed to be getting rid of. If you reinforce your case with the help of your mate, this will make it *more stuck* and you have the likelihood of getting *more sick*.

The same is true vice versa...your colluding with them could make them more sick. In the book *Love Without Conditions*, my friend Paul Ferrini calls this "The Tyranny of Agreement." In other words, the ego cannot conceive that there is any love when two people disagree. If you are supporting behavior that could be hurtful to your mate, this is the ultimate codependency. Peace does not come through the agreement of two egos. The truly "healthy" relationship has room for disagreement. One can even disagree without upsets. If one listens carefully to a mate who is disagreeing, then one can learn what one needs to change in order to stay healthy.

Married couples often tend to think they have to back their spouse no matter what. But what if your spouse is out of integrity? Well, if you are supporting that kind of thing, then you are not only colluding, you are adding to your own karma!

So then, where is the balance? How do you support a mate without supporting his or her ego? And how can one handle this without making them feel that they are wrong and that you are being too critical? Ah, very good question! I have tried to address this in my recent book, *ESSAYS ON CREATING SACRED RELATION-SHIPS -THE NEW PARADIGM.* It has to do with knowing what is real and what is the ego. Then, handling that well, it has to do with attitude, grace, enlightenment, and excellent communication skills. Now we are talking about the dynamics of a relationship. Now we are talking about the real *art* of creating a relationship with good dynamics. If you truly love your mate, you do not support his or her case, nor make it real, nor allow him to get by with it. Instead you provide the safety, the love, tenderness and kindness for this person to feel safe enough to look at what they are doing to themselves.

You are the mirror, and you offer them a new turn that would be healthier for them than the one they are taking. But you would have to ever-so-gently first help them to see that the way they are going now may hurt them or others. If you point that out in a harsh way, they will, however feel hurt by you, and they will resist.

When, however, you face the fact that you are the one you live with, you will see that it is also you out there you are talking to. (Why do *you* have this situation in *your* vibration?) Your mate you are upset with is *your* mirror. What they are doing is probably something that was done in your childhood that you need to forgive. Ultimately, working on your own case is the answer; and being willing to get help with that is a good idea. Tell your mate that you actually want him or her to point out to you when you are off. Who wants a "yes man" anyway? How boring!! (Only someone who is totally insecure.)

Try this attitude: Welcome criticism. Be glad when someone points out your faults. They are healing you. This surely is a big opportunity for you to grow. Welcome feedback. It is good for you. If people are fabricating things about you, insulting you, or inappropriately abusing you, you should be unshakable even then and not let it ruffle you. But of course, you should look to see how you attracted *that* and try to keep from attracting that result ever again. My guru Babaji said to us, "Be not concerned with praise or abuse...do your work!" This advice has helped me so many times as a leader.

I have known many married couples whom I also knew pretty well as single people before they had met each other. Before they met, they were each very strong in their own right, with tremendous potential, often making great contributions. However, a while after moving in with each other, they more or less "caved in" on each other and became dependent and weak. Often they "sold out" and gave up dreams and did not become at all what they could have been. I often saw them almost destroying each other. Why?? The answer is a long one. I wrote the whole LRT training in an attempt to answer that one.

Obviously, the point is that a relationship should strengthen one - not weaken one. You should be happier because of the relationship, not more miserable. You should *expand* because of the relationship, not contract. You should get financially more prosperous as a result, not less. You should get healthier, not sicker. This is the goal, the ideal. However, in order to handle everything that comes up in a relationship, and to keep growing stronger, enlightenment is required. Instead of saying it feels impossible, try reading the *Course In Miracles* and see why the above is not happening for you.

If your mate does happen to become ill, the way you handle that also affects the outcome. If you go into agreement with the illness and make it real and give it undue attention, you are both reinforcing it. If you start feeling very sorry for your mate, and worrying, and treating him like an invalid, you are only making it worse. That does not mean you are to be "cold" and ignore someone who needs support. The support they need may not be what you thought, however.

Encouragement and love without making someone more helpless is a good start!

It is best to see them as "healed". Keep imagining them without the condition and help them heal by using the techniques in this book. Your confidence in a miraculous outcome can make a difference that is huge. I KNOW it is hard when you are in love with the person and you are panicked, thinking that they might abandon you by dying or something. Perhaps you will need help yourself in order to hold the highest thought.

One of the main ways you can support someone who has become ill is to make sure they do not forget to do the truth process just as soon as they get symptoms. Do not to wait until they get a full blown illness with a major "diagnosis". Also study the *CIM* pamphlets which explain how Jesus healed people. Try to align with HIS MIND. Where would I be today if people had gone into agreement with my arthritis? I would not be writing this book, probably.

I know many people that are staying in destructive or dead relationships because they are too afraid to leave. Staying in a relationship because you are too afraid to leave is not a good reason for staying. And is it even ethical? If you are lying to yourself and being unethical in your staying, your chances for getting sick are greater.

People often ask me if they should leave a relationship now or wait and see if it ever clears up. This is not for me to decide. What I do tell them is to pray for this relationship to be healed, OR for something better for both of them. That way, either way it is a win. I tell them to pray for *Divine Right Action*. Of course, there are many cases in which conditions suddenly shifted and miracles happened. Of course, we all know of cases in which people stayed too long and they totally regretted it. I know that one must pray a lot on these points.

Just the other day I received a letter from a woman who wrote, "It is strange how I have been hanging on to this extremely painful relationship; and now I feel *so relieved* that it is over. I am like a new person." (As for me, I know if I had stayed in my first marriage, I would likely be sick right now and there would have been no LRT.)

And then, miracles can happen even in the cases of the worst scenarios. This takes two persons' total commitment. And the only way to have a perfect relationship is to have both people willing to experience their own perfection. So I would say that commitment to self-improvement and spiritual enlightenment has to be the top priority for both, in order for the healing of the relationship to happen. Denying and pretending will only be destructive to the body.

Some relationships have been destroyed because the couple never learned good communication habits. There is a vast area for improvement in this area for all of us. It is worth spending the time to study effective communication. I know I could have stayed longer in some relationships if I had known how to communicate better.

Influence of Communication

What you are *not* saying could be making you sick or keeping you in pain. Werner Erhard, the founder of EST, used to say to us, "What you cannot communicate runs you." Well, I was always a very talkative person and after I heard that, I talked even more! However, I wondered, was it *true* communication? Was I really saying my truest feelings? I began saying them more. I began really telling people what I wanted and what I thought. That appeared to be working. Then I began writing. This form of expression helped me even more. I thought, "Oh, boy! I am really expressing myself well." I thought I was on top of it. But I was not really.

The next level was having to face what I was in denial about and admit that. That was scarier. It was shocking to me to find out that there were things I was afraid to say. It all came to a head on a trip to Australia where I had some trouble with my hip. A guide told me that I was now starting to process genetic ancestral material. Then she shocked me by proceeding to tell me that my grandparents from Sweden, long ago dead, had appeared to her. They wanted me to know that there was a big secret in my family, and she even told me what it was. I was stunned, but I knew it was true because right away it kind of explained a whole section of our family life which I had never been able to understand. She told me it would take several months to process that family pattern.

Well, I wanted to speed things up, so I had some cranial-osteo work in Spain by Geraldine. She intuitively worked on my gums one whole hour. Then she told me some anger would come out and I would no longer be able to withhold anything; and I would get out of denial about many things that I needed to communicate. But I *still* did not think I had anything to communicate that was so big. I was really unable to see it. But within the next few days it all came out. I knew suddenly whom I had to communicate with and what I had to communicate about. But it was still scary. I thought there would be anger. I was so afraid of anger that to keep peace I was withholding a lot of stuff. So then I was faced with how to communicate this delicate material which was truly affecting my business. Very tricky. First I had to write copious faxes about my fear of communicating. Then I spent days being "very diplomatic". Then one day I was not so diplomatic. It was rocky. I hung in there. After all this I felt much, much better physically. My energy went way up in my body. There was a dramatic increase in my power and happiness. But I should have done it long ago before it had become so hard to make changes. I waited far too long. My business was "sick" by then.

Maybe you are sick or in pain because you are too afraid to say to your mate, "Today I really feel like leaving this relationship." There is a great chance that if you just say it and you feel heard, your desire to leave will also change.

I have heard of a number of cases in which people finally began communicating something to a person in the family - when that person was on the death bed! I guess the feeling was: "Well since he is going to die anyway, this cannot kill him." I know of a guy who finally told his mother, as she lay dying, something that she had done that had really bothered him his whole life. She was so sorry he had not told her sooner because the whole thing was a complete misunderstanding, a communication problem. She had meant it just the opposite of the way he took it. The incident had been affecting his whole life negatively for nearly 40 years. Problems are started by poor communication, but then you need good communication to clear up the problems.

For years in our community, we tried the way of *Direct Feedback*. This was an overcompensation for withholds. This was better than "stuffing it", but I kept noticing that people still got on the defensive unless the feedback was worded perfectly. The person receiving the feedback often felt attacked and instead of really hearing the communication, began to find a way to attack back by similarly strong feedback. We plowed through this and we got better at it. Better at giving it and better at receiving it. I prided myself at being able to "take criticism". I felt I had enough self-esteem. But I never felt satisfied with the whole thing because for many it was too devastating.

I also noticed that for the really delicate, hard, sensitive things that people were still afraid to say, they would tell someone else rather than the "offending" person directly. Then this would get back to the person it was really intended for. That person would call up and confront the one who had said it to someone else. The person who had said it would deny it, back down, or usually say, "Oh, I did not mean it that way at all. So-and-so misunderstood." This drove me nuts. I tried to give a lecture on all this to the community at a summer event. But I saw little change that year.

Then I read an article about some group in San Diego studying communication. A man had developed what he called compassionate communication. He recommended that one say:

1) "What I feel is...
"

2) "What I want is..
"

Example:
"What I feel is sad because I cannot get this issue about the children resolved."

"What I want is a resolution by tomorrow night. So I need for you to think about it and tell me your desired result by then." Instead of, "You don't handle this issue about the children. You never deal with it at all. You avoid everything. I don't think you are a good father and you don't support me!"

It is really important to hear out everyone in a family and relationship. Give them space to say everything without interruptions. Then say, "THANK YOU" instead of being on the defensive. This discharges the energy and they will be able to drop the upset. You will be surprised how much better you will feel physically after these simple procedures.

Another good thing to remember is that when a person is upset and coming at you, it is best to just listen and then see if you can find one thing you agree with. You might not agree with most of it, but start out by saying :

"I can see your point about.............................."

"I agree with.............................."

Then stop to integrate this alignment.

Try reading the book *You Just Don't Understand* to learn more about the differences in male and female communication. Also I have written more on this in the book *VIBRATING TO THE NEW PARADIGM.*

Part IV

Methods of Spiritual Healing

Spiritual Healing Techniques

The following is a method of healing I have developed over years and years of study. It is so simple that now I wonder why it has taken me so long to get it. Perhaps it was because it has taken me a long time to unravel my addiction to Western medicine, and that had to go out first. Then I had to integrate all my years of Rebirthing, training in India and what the *Course in Miracles* says. After that I kind of "reduced it all down" like a sauce.

There are 3 main parts to this Self-Healing Technique:

I. FINDING THE CAUSE OF THE CONDITION (The REAL cause...the metaphysical cause.)

II. CONFESSION OF THE ADDICTION (The addiction to those negative thoughts causing the condition.)

III. SPIRITUAL PURIFICATION METHODS (For releasing the thoughts that cause the condition.)

I. FINDING THE CAUSE: This is accomplished through what I call the "Ultimate Truth Process" which can be done in writing. In this way you become your own Sherlock Holmes and you tell the absolute truth to yourself on paper. You must let go of the thought, "I don't know", because that will block your ability to access the information. You DO know the cause of your condition. It is in your mind. You just have to let the responses come up to consciousness. A writing process helps you do that. On paper you write the following:

A. *The negative thoughts I have that are causing this condition are:*

B. *My "payoffs" for having this condition are:*

C. *My fears of giving up this condition are:*

D. *My most negative thought about my body is:*

E. *My most negative thought about myself is:*

F. *When this condition first began was:*

G. *What was going on in my life at that time was....*

See next page for an example of this truth process. This technique is called "Self-Analysis".

II. CONFESSION: Recognizing the above data as an addiction (something I am stubbornly hanging on to) I confess to God and another person that I am indulging regularly in the above ego thoughts and I have been refusing to let go of them. (Read to another person the above list you have written and, standing before your altar, read it to the Holy Spirit.)

III. SPIRITUAL PURIFICATION METHODS:

Some examples are:
Affirmations
Prayer
Rebirthing
Chanting
Meditation
Fasting
Indian Sweat Lodges
Writing
Silence...Seclusion
Visiting an Ashram
Head Shaving.

(See my book *Pure Joy* for the other methods and all explanations.)

REALITY CHECK
It is good to have a buddy who also understands these techniques to do a reality check with you. The ideal reality check person would be your personal Rebirther.

Another process you can do with your Rebirther or buddy is a verbal truth process such as this: The following is a "Sentence Completion Technique".

"I will allow myself to be healed when ...."

Keep repeating this phrase and fill in the blank. We are not talking about a time span here. You are confessing to your buddy what you think needs to happen before you are safe enough to let go of the condition.

Example:
"I will be healed of....................(when I am sure my mother is okay first.)"

"I will allow myself to be healed of..................(when I feel I have suffered enough over my sister's death.)"

"I will allow myself to be healed of......................(when I experience my perfection.)"

A skilled Rebirther would then take you deeper and have you say:

"I will know my mother is okay when...................."

"I will feel I have suffered enough when................"

"I will experience my perfection when...................."

These "answers" will give the Rebirther necessary information about why you are not allowing yourself to be healed NOW. Sometimes you may be setting up for yourself impossible situations, such as "I cannot let myself be healed because my mother is not healed." Well, maybe your mother, brother or family member does not want to be healed and you will therefore have to wait forever. Waiting for family members to go first is a mistake. You go first and set an example. The Rebirther will help you process and breathe out unrealistic expectations.

Here is an example of the Ultimate Truth Process (writing):

Condition - *Extremely Dry Skin*

1. *The thoughts causing this condition are*:
a. I don't drink enough water.
b. A part of me is "dead".
c. I want to be like my grandmother.
d. I don't want to be too seductive.
e. I don't want to be touched too much.
f. The exact negative thought causing this condition is that I can be more like a man and be like my father.

2. *My payoffs for having this condition are*:
a. I don't have to be too feminine.
b. I can keep men away.
c. I don't have to be too sensual.
d. My biggest pay off for having this condition is that I don't have to be seductive.

3. *My fears of giving up this condition are*:
a. With beautiful skin, I would seduce men more and have to be a real woman. (My father wants a boy, not a girl.)
b. I would have more sex and more touching and I would be distracted by that.
c. I would attract too many people if I were totally radiant.
d. My biggest fear of giving up this condition is that I would be glowing and saint-like. I am afraid of perfection.

My most negative thought about my body is that it won't do what I want.

My most negative thought about myself is I am not perfect.

This condition started when??? Teenage, when my father died.

I want to say a few more words to explain the meaning of "payoff". A "payoff" is something that one is getting out of a condition that is neurotic or something negative that one is trying to "prove".

If the "payoff" is too great, the person may not want to give up the condition. Furthermore, in order to give up the condition, one has to be willing to also give up the "payoffs". Therefore it is important to not only to understand what the payoffs are, but it is even more important to learn that one does not need these neurotic payoffs. Below I am listing some more examples of payoffs.

Note that the word "symptom" is interchangeable with "disease".

Typical Payoffs for keeping symptoms or diseases:

Attention.

Punishing oneself with the condition because of guilt.

Keeping people away.

Using the symptom to prove that one is helpless, bad, worthless, unable, not perfect, not good enough, a failure, etc.

Punishing a mate or parent to try to make them feel that they are not good enough or are bad.

Using the symptoms as a way of holding oneself back because of fear of moving forward.

Using the symptom as a form of conflict because one is addicted to conflict.

Using the symptom as a way of trying to prove that there is no God.

Using the symptom as an excuse to be angry.

Using the symptom as an excuse not to work.

Using the symptom or disease as a cover up or distraction to avoid what is really going on.

Using the symptom as a way of sabotaging one's life, career or relationship.

Using the symptom as a way of deadening oneself because of fear of feeling and/or fear of life.

There are healthier, less neurotic ways to handle these issues. For example, you don't have to be sick to get attention. You can learn that self-punishment in the form of sickness is not necessary. You could forgive yourself instead. You could change jobs and find something you love to do rather than getting sick to get out of a job you hate, etc. You can actually leave a relationship' instead of getting sick to get out of it.

Examples of FEARS people might have about giving up the disease or symptom:

Fear that if one gave it up, one might have to be responsible.

Fear that if one should give it up, one might have to succeed.

Fear that if one should give it up, one might have to face something.

Fear that if one should give it up, one might have to move forward and be powerful.

Fear that if one should give it up, one could no longer get even.

Fear that if one should give it up, one would have no more excuses.

Fear that if one should give it up, one might have to be happy.

Fear that if one should give it up, one might end up with a relationship and then one would have to handle love.

Fear that if one should give it up, one might end up alone.

You may *think* you do not have any fear of giving up the condition; but if you still have the condition, then you still have the fear. When you work out the fear, you will be ready to give up the condition. (See section on fear of healing under the *Course In Miracles* section.) So the first step is to identify the fear, and the next step is to give up the fear. Change the thoughts that cause the fear and breathe out the feeling of fear.

Prayers for Healing

I am quite willing to share with you the prayers I use for healing, but I do feel that you ultimately should work out your own so that they have more personal meaning to you. It took me a number of years to get this right for myself. For one thing, in order for me to get "back into" prayer, I had to work out my case with religion and all my disappointment around religious theology. After leaving the church, rebelling and then reentering spirituality through Rebirthing, I had to find my way again.

When I met my guru Babaji, he allowed me to write to him all my prayers in the form of letters. I decided that one purpose of a guru was to permit you to bare your soul to him. So that is what I did. I would share with him all my problems, lay them at his feet, and ask for guidance. Usually I would have an "emotional release" during this process and my energy would shift. Then I would experience a change in my body. I actually did this for years...but now when I think of it, these prayers seem kind of crude and embarrassing to me. But in a sense it was the best I could do and was my way of "giving it to the Holy Spirit". Later, after Babaji entered his final Samadhi, I continued to write him and still do to this day. I place the prayers on my altar until I feel the issue clears. It STILL works for me. But now it works better because I have learned to compose the prayers in a more responsible way.

First I state my gratitude and forgiveness.
Then I state my problem.
Then I try to confess how I created this problem myself -
what ego thoughts, negative thoughts of mine were in operation.
Then I lay those at his feet.
Then I ask for the ability to see the problem differently.
Then I choose new thinking to counteract my old thoughts.
Then I ask to have the new positive thinking fortified.

In this way, I am taking more responsibility for my case and showing the Divine that I am willing to do something about it. *I am not saying, "Oh, please do it for me."* Begging for something is a lower form of prayer. Gratitude is the highest form of prayer.

Sometimes I add other steps. I sit before my altar and speak aloud to Babaji, Jesus, the Divine Mother, etc....all of whom represent the Holy Spirit's mind to me. At first I felt silly doing this and really embarrassed. But the results were fantastic, so I went ahead anyway. The desire to communicate with the Masters is essential to opening the door to their presence. It must start with you. You have to **INVITE IN** the Holy Spirit.

There is a five-part prayer I learned as a child in the Lutheran Church which is really excellent:

1. *Opening*
2. *Forgiveness*
3. *Gratitude*
4. *Petition*
5. *Closing*

1. OPENING: In this part you "set the state" and get into the proper frame of mind. This I do by repeating mantras or by reading from *A Course In Miracles* workbook the lesson for today. You could also read from the Bible or from any spiritual metaphysical book that is important to you.

2. FORGIVENESS: In this step you state the following:
a. What you want to be forgiven for.
b. Whom you want to be forgiven by.
c. Whom you want to forgive, etc.

3. GRATITUDE:
Now you state, with deep feeling, everything that you are grateful for and everybody you are grateful to, with love and appreciation.

4. PETITION: At this point you actually ask for guidance and help with specific problems. (Here I would read specific prayers for healing of the body...see example below.)

5. CLOSING: Finally you again read the scriptures. The *Course In Miracles* text would be ideal.

Example of #4, Petition: You would read this at your altar:
Regarding my condition of gastritis (for example):
"I take responsibility for creating this condition caused by the negative thoughts of mine such as..................."

"I lay this at your feet. I allow you, the Holy Spirit, to

undo all my wrong thinking that caused this condition and those thoughts that keep me from giving it up." (Read the negative thoughts from your truth process as a confession.)

"I now choose to think that I can create PEACE instead of this. I place it all in your hands. I ask you to help release me from this and raise it from me."

"I ask to be taught the right perception of the body."

"I pray for release from the *fear* of the miracle healing. I pray for help in the cause of that *fear*, which is my addiction to the thought of separation from God."

"I DO NOT WANT TO KEEP THIS ERROR."

"I now ask (the part of the body affected...in this case, intestines) to cooperate and let go. I cooperate with You and follow You. (The Mind of Jesus.) I believe that You know what to do and will guide me. I choose union with you. I am willing to receive the solution."

"I have total willingness to have God's Will for me which is Perfect Happiness and Perfect Health. I know that in You, in your mercy and WILL that I will be saved from this."

"I therefore completely release the thought that this cannot be healed. The completed results of Jesus Christ now manifest for me in this situation. This is the time for Divine Completion!"

If the above prayer does not produce results, try this one:

Begin by placing your palms down as a symbolic indication of your willingness and desire to turn over any concerns you may have to God. Examples:

Say :
"Lord, I give you my anger at.............................."
(palms down)   (palms down)"

"Lord, I would like to receive your divine love for ...." (palms up)

"Lord, I release my fear of never being healed of ...." (palms down)

"Lord, I receive now your certainty that I can be healed of.........................." (palms up)

"Lord, I surrender my anxiety about my weight and body." (palms down)

"Lord, I receive now your peace about my weight and body." (palms up)

When you do these hands-down and hands-up movements, spend some minutes in complete silence and wait until you feel something. Do not rush this process. Allow God to Commune with your Spirit.

Note: Prayer *does* have the power to heal. Scientific studies actually prove it. Dr. Larry Dossey, Co- Chairman of the National Institutes for Health has reported many studies in which patients have responded remarkably to prayer. In fact, prayed-for patients were five times less likely to develop complications or need antibiotics. So if you are very ill, not only should you try the prayers above, but why not get yourself on a prayer list and let people pray for you? It works.

Rebirthing and Healing

Rebirthing, or Conscious Breathing, is a physical, mental, and spiritual experience. The physical part consists of connecting your inhale and exhale in a relaxed rhythm. (No holding at the top or bottom.) The spiritual dimension of conscious breathing is the heart of the matter. One of the purposes of Rebirthing is not only the movement of air, but the movement of *energy.* The dynamic "energy flows" that are experienced when Rebirthing are the merging of Spirit and matter. The "energy flows" are the process of filling your body with pure life-energy and cleaning your mind and body of tension and impurities. You can also remember and release your birth trauma in Rebirthing, and this makes a huge difference in your life. There is dry Rebirthing and wet Rebirthing. It should always be conducted by a well-trained Rebirther. (See appendix for information on locating one in your area.) Only after one has become a Rebirther and has passed certain levels of expertise should one try to Rebirth oneself.

This kind of conscious breathing gives you a great self-healing power! We think of Rebirthing as the ultimate healing experience because your breath, together with the quality of your thoughts, can heal you rapidly. We have seen symptoms, from migraine headaches to ulcers to sore ankles, disappear completely as a result of Rebirthing. Respiratory illnesses, stomach and back pains have disappeared. Frigidity, hemorrhoids, insomnia, diabetes, epilepsy, cancer, arthritis, and all kinds of other manifestations have been eliminated. Many of these conditions seem to have been caused or pro-longed by birth traumas. Leonard Orr, the founder of Rebirthing, said, "People get stuck in birth trauma symptoms and then develop medical belief symptoms about them." He added, "Doctors can then become mother substitutes to support infancy patterns."

In Rebirthing, we see people go through physiological changes in ten minutes that other people stay stuck in for years and from which they may even die.

On the other hand, Rebirthing creates a safe environment in your mind and body for symptoms from the past, such as childhood illnesses and patterns, to act themselves out. It is a good idea to keep in mind that these symptoms are temporary and relatively easy to eliminate with uninhibited breathing. (Some people have created diaper rash for example.) But if, in your mind, you are afraid of childhood symptoms or resent them, you may inhibit your natural healing powers.

If you have a lot of fear, it is a good idea to consult physicians that you really trust, as well as spiritual and mental healers, until you work out the fear of self-healing. They will help you get out of the traps in your mind.

Rebirthing is not for people who retreat from life in fear or who desire to curl up and die - unless they want to retreat from that pattern! Rebirthing is for people who desire to live fully, freely, and healthfully in Spirit, Mind and Body. We do not claim that any cure is permanent because human beings have the power to recreate any symptoms. But *Permanent Healing* IS the goal and IS available. However, it is up to the individual to accept the opportunity.

Rebirthing creates a safe environment in the mind and body which enables clients to become free of all negativity; however, processing negativity can be overwhelming at times. That is why we recommend you take it gently and start out with only one session a week. We also recommend that you make the whole process of spiritual growth easier by participating in a spiritual community that assists you effectively and supports you in whatever changes you may go through. Cultivating the philosophy of Physical Immortality also gives you optimism, and makes conquering all difficulties an adventure instead of a bewildering tragedy.

I could have presented many examples of healing by Rebirthing. Obviously, many volumes would be required to relate the complexities of all the personal case histories of people we have helped. But even if you labored through them, they still might not help you. There is really no substitute for trusting your own intuition about your body and with a community of friends who can add their wisdom to your personal healing.

The purpose of Rebirthing actually was not for healing in the beginning, but healing turned out to be a valuable by-product. The purpose of Rebirthing is to acquaint people with a dimension of spiritual energy which they may not have heretofore experienced. When people are experiencing this process, they are able to connect their illness or pain with the original negative thought out of which it was created, and thereby take total responsibility for causing it. Some people are therefore completely able to let go of the condition instantaneously during the session. It literally gets pumped out of the body with the breath. Others may let go of it gradually during the following weeks after the session. The breath is the cleanser of the body, as the yogis have always known.

It is usually possible to come out of Rebirthing in a perpetual state of health and bliss, but the path could be rocky. For example, when people experience their actual birth in Rebirthing, they may also go into re-experiencing various stages of infancy and some feelings of helplessness. In my own Rebirthing, I noticed that I never went through something I could not handle; the harder things came up only when I was strong enough to take it. But these rocky periods did not bother me because the more I worked out my birth trauma, the more energy I experienced. And this kept increasing and still is. For the rocky parts, I was able to remember that "This will pass". Also, Rebirthing ultimately raises your self-esteem; when that happens, all areas of your life are affected positively.

People may avoid Rebirthing because they experience fear when they even hear the word! It is not that Rebirthing *adds* to your fear however. One of the purposes of Rebirthing is to *release* fear. Feeling fear when you think of Rebirthing just shows you how much fear you have suppressed in your body since day one. Just the word Rebirthing stimulates that fear. Breathing it out will be a great relief. I personally would never commit my life to something that was dangerous. I have learned that it is more dangerous to keep the birth trauma suppressed in oneself.

The following information is taken from the book *Rebirthing in the New Age* which I wrote with Leonard Orr, the founder of Rebirthing.

"The birth trauma is your introduction to the world. It is the beginning of the "The Universe is Against Me" syndrome. There are preverbal thoughts and there is preverbal intelligence. Your thinking began before you were able to verbalize those thoughts - in other words, before you were born. Therefore, when you were born, you were able to make sophisticated conclusions about that traumatic event. The womb is a comfortable place where all physiological needs are supplied. When we are pulled from this ideal environment, we experience a considerable amount of pain and discomfort. Probably 90% of our fear originated with the birth trauma. Some of the generalizations we might have made at birth are:

"Being outside of the womb is unpleasant."
"I cannot trust people."
"If this is what life is like, I don't want to be here."
"People are out to get me."
"I can't get enough air (love), nourishment, etc."

"The birth trauma is one of the reasons most people don't like to get up in the morning. The bed simulates the womb experience. In the process of awakening, the memory of birth pains are stimulated to near-consciousness. These near-memories trigger the fear that you will have to re-experience being born again. Warm baths and showers also stimulate womb experiences. (Some people choose even a hospital as a substitute for the womb or Heaven.) Even something like smoking can symbolize being back in the womb...trying to get to the comfort of having the lungs full as they were in the womb."

"Impatience, hostility and susceptibility to illness and accidents can sometimes be traced back to the birth trauma. Many people feel either too hot or too cold and never experience lasting physical comfort during their entire lifetimes because of unpleasant birth experiences. We view the traditional theological description of Heaven as a symbolic description of the womb. What people are really after when they seek "Heaven" is to get back to that feeling of the womb. People want to go back to the womb because it has not been very pleasant since they came out; and it is unpleasant because of the negative decisions they made at birth, which produce negative results. The Rebirthing experience was created to enable you to go back and dissolve all that."

Other Alternatives

EMOTIONAL RELEASE:

Usually I have found that when I need to let go of any stubborn pattern or symptom, I need to let myself break down and cry at some point in order to get the physical release.

Of course, this is easier to do during Rebirthing. Having a Rebirther present to keep you breathing through it, helps the energy move. If I do not have a fellow Rebirther, I can usually get myself to cry by Wet Rebirthing myself in the bathtub. However I do NOT recommend that you try it on your own until you have reached a certain point in the Rebirthing Process and your Rebirther, having trained you, feels you are ready. I point it out, however, as it is something to work towards and look forward to.

There are other ways to get oneself to cry and have an emotional release. I can make myself "crack" also by throwing myself face down completely on the floor in front of my altar and repenting my mistakes. Another way I do it, is to lie down on the bed and talking aloud to Jesus until I finally let go and cry.

Since I am a writer, the fastest thing for me to do is to write to my guru Babaji and confess my case on paper. You do not have to be a professional writer to write a confession to God. Usually when I get down to the bottom line, I start crying. This cleansing always works for me.

Another thing one can do is sit across from a friend

and say, "Something I feel sad about is...." "Another thing I feel sad about is...." If one is getting down to the bottom line and telling the *real* truth, usually the sadness will finally manifest in tears and you will feel better. You can often heal yourself of symptoms by having a very deep crying session (especially symptoms of cold and sinus).

The point is that not only does one have to change one's thoughts to be healed, but it is of particular importance to breathe out the negative mental mass. Feeling the feeling is also part of this process. Feeling fear and sadness rather than stuffing it is one of the secrets of staying healthy. I may be crying because I am sad about a situation, but I also cry often as a way of repenting my mistakes. It is humbling to feel the sadness of one's errors. It helps me to admit to God aloud that I have been wrong in my thinking (which is obvious or I would not have the symptom). If you are not feeling well, you have chosen wrongly.

To some people it might seem easier to just go to a doctor and get some pills. But, believe me, pills are only temporary relief. If you don't get the consciousness factor that causes your symptoms, the symptoms can easily return, possibly in a worse form. *The Course In Miracles* says that pills are forms of "spell". They work if you *believe* they work, but putting a "spell" on yourself like that does not work in the long run. Pills, ultimately, are not needed if you surrender to the healing power of God. However, on certain occasions, if you have too much fear of spiritual healing, you should not judge yourself if you take a medical treatment. But the goal should be to eventually wean yourself of that. Feeling your emotions and releasing them is one of the keys.

MOVEMENT:

Sometimes it helps to say prayers and mantras with movement, especially if you can walk on the beach or on a relatively quiet path. It is very good to play a tape of mantras and walk very fast while repeating them. This really moves the energy in your body and cracks your case. I find it much more interesting and effective than gymnastic workouts.

If you ever feel too sick or out-of-it to walk fast, move, or even chant, at least put the earphones on your head with the mantras playing as loudly as you can stand and prostrate yourself in front of the altar even if you have to crawl to get there. That is a symbolic "movement" of humility.

I hope that you will call your Rebirther before you get too sick. By the way, if you have symptoms, don't cancel your Rebirthing appointment! That is the exact time you need to go. GET MOVING toward your Rebirther.

Another form of movement that you can do that is not too overwhelming when you have symptoms is this: Put on some music of African drums. Just stand in place and shake your body. Close your eyes and don't worry about how you look. Keep doing this and then lie down and breathe with your Rebirther. Your breathing mechanism will be more open and productive as a result of that simple movement.

If you find exercise too strenuous and inappropriate because you are feeling too awful, maybe you should follow your intuition and not force yourself. Perhaps something as simple as the above will get you started. Then later you could try something else nice like sacred dance or an activity that has meaning for you.

Recently I have experimented with Watsu Therapy, movement done under water. I have found this to be *very* effective. I recommend it strongly as a healing technique. Watsu therapy is a healing art, and because of the water, the body can easily assume positions that would be very difficult to assume outside the water. The spinal fluid is stimulated in such a way that the natural healing powers of the body are enhanced. The therapy requires minimal effort because the Watsu therapist is in charge of moving your body. So you could really be feeling helpless and still get the benefit of the movements. After the session you most likely will feel like moving again by yourself. It is a nice transition. Often when you feel sick, the last thing you want to do is move even though it might help. In this case, the resistance is handled because the Watsu therapist knows how to move you, and the positions are not hard to assume under the water.

For information, contact Two Bunch Palms Resort in Palm Springs, California or Harbon Hot Springs, California.

Diet, Health and Healing

There are so many opinions on this subject that one could easily read one hundred different books and get one hundred different opinions. You can feel crazy after a while, trying to figure it all out. For me, one of the hardest things in my life that I had to work out for myself was the subject of health and nutrition. That was because:
a) I was born on the kitchen table.
b) I was born in the food belt of the world.
c) My mother was a home economics teacher and I had to learn innumerable "rules" about food that were supposed to make me healthy.

In the end I rebelled against all of it because I felt that I was going mad. I had to write the book *The Only Diet There Is* to heal myself so that I could relax even enough to eat at all. I had been so obsessed with this subject for so many years that I had tried too many different "diets", too many different ways of eating, too many food plans, too many nutrition programs, too many nutrition products. *Too* many to even think straight.

And in the end, I reduced it down to the fact that I *like* being a vegetarian. It feels right to me physically, morally and energetically. I also like the results. And yet that is just another opinion: MINE! You have to find out what works for you. I have been a vegetarian well over a decade and it makes me happy. Once a year, I try to eat a hot dog so I am not rigid. But now that is getting hard to do.

I honestly feel the whole subject is best summed up by another fellow Immortalist, JoAnna Cherry. She expresses my sincerest feelings even better than I can. This particular paragraph is from the chapter called *Divine Self* in the book *New Cells, New Bodies, New Life,* by Virginia Essene and others. I recommend this book, obviously.

"Are you eating what feels most right for you at this time? Foods are all thought forms, just like our body; and we do have the ability to transform any food - with our thought, love, light, intention - to a frequency that is totally beneficial to our body. But until we fully empower ourselves with this ability, our body will love some food more than others. Raw and organic fruits and vegetables, soaked nuts and sprouted seeds and beans hold the greatest natural light. Many wonderful new substances are available today also that can enliven and lift your body. Try and just listen to your Spirit and the highest desire for your body, and follow that."

I have discussed this topic more fully in the book *The Only Diet There Is,* which teaches you how to keep the weight you want by the power of your mind, and also in my book on Physical Immortality, *How To Be Chic, Fabulous, and Live Forever.* In that book I discussed some of the research on which diets are believed to enhance longevity.

On the subject of vegetarianism, again, there are certain Immortal teachers who say that if you eat meat, you are participating in the karma of killing, and this does not cooperate with your desire to be Immortal. But, the *other* argument is that that is just another thought which you could change! So, you see, you just have to think for yourself. You do have to determine whether or not your thoughts are powerful enough to overcome these aspects; you have to decide how you feel morally, etc.

You might need to consider this: If your thoughts were clear enough, you could drink even poison and not die. (But would you test this out?????) Kahuna Masters have done that. I have met one. But most of us don't go around testing this. We don't go around proving we can drink poison. Well, then, are we ready and able to process poisonous food? Why make it hard for yourself? Also, which foods do you think are poisonous? Maybe everyone should actually read *Diet for a New America.* When you read that and find out what *really goes on* when meat and poultry are processed, you might not feel like eating any of it again. One should investigate all this for oneself and decide for oneself. I would not recommend that you rely on what you were taught in school on this subject! How do you know that that was the highest thought? It probably was not. Nor do I want to insist that my opinion is the right one.

I do have to admit, however, that I have been influenced somewhat by great minds who wrote about these subjects. Here are some examples:

JESUS: "And the flesh of slain beasts in his body will become his own tomb. For I tell you truly, he who kills, kills himself; and who so eats the flesh of slain beasts eats the body of death."

BUDDHA: "Let the Bodhisattva who is disciplining himself to attain compassion refrain from eating flesh. Meat is food for ferocious beasts: improper to eat...so said the Buddha. If, bereft of compassion and wisdom, you eat meat, you have turned your back on liberation."

DA VINCI, LEONARDO: "Truly, man is the king of beasts, for his brutality exceeds theirs. We live by the death of others. We are burial places. The time will come when men such as I will look upon the murder of animals as they now look upon the murder of men."

SHELLY, PERCY BYSSHE: "It is only by softening and disguising dead flesh by culinary preparation that it is rendered susceptible of mastication or digestion, and that the sight of its bloods, juices and red horror does not excite intolerable loathing and disgust. Let the advocate of animal food force himself to a decisive experiment of its fitness and, as Plutarch recommends, tear a living lamb with his teeth and, plunging his head into its vitals, slake his thirst with the steaming blood. When fresh from the deed of horror, let him revert to the irresistible instincts of nature that would rise in judgment against it, and say, 'Nature forced me for such work as this.' Then, and then only, would he be consistent."

THOREAU, HENRY: "I have no doubt that it is part of the destiny of the human race, in its gradual development, to leave off the eating of animals as surely as the savage tribes have left off eating each other when they came into contact with the more civilized."

TOLSTOY, LEO: "Vegetarianism serves as a criterion by which we know that the pursuit of moral perfection on the path of man is genuine and sincere. It is dreadful that man suppresses in himself, unnecessarily, the highest spiritual capacity...that of sympathy and pity towards living creatures like himself... and by violating his own feelings becomes cruel. And how deeply seated in the human heart is the injunction not to take life."

BESANT, ANNIE: "People who eat meat are responsible for all the pain that grows out of meat eating, and which is necessitated by the use of sentient animals as food...not only the horrors of the slaughterhouse, but all the preliminary horrors of railway or ship traffic, all the starvation and the thirst and the prolonged misery of fear which these unhappy creatures have to pass through for the gratification of the appetite of men. All pain acts as a record against humanity and slackens and retards the whole of human growth."

I was quite glad that I was a vegetarian myself before I found this book. I do admit that this book influenced me to stay with it. Notice if what they said makes you angry. If you are still a meat eater, it might make you angry. Just look at that. These great minds would probably propose that your anger is a result of eating meat! Well, just remember that the book is called *Food for Thought*. Please do not invalidate my whole book just because you might be angry at these quotes. I did not say that you *have to* give up meat. I am merely saying that it is a good idea to think it over and be really clear on your decision. What might happen is that you might realize that you have been brainwashed by school, parents, TV and nutritionists. Maybe you have never considered your own spiritual feelings. Maybe you have never tried to be a vegetarian and maybe you would like it. Who knows? As for me, I prayed about it. I said, "If this is right, take the desire for meat from me. I am willing for Divine Right Action." I left Bali and did not want red meat or poultry after that.

I have been discussing food from a standpoint of health maintenance. It is also true that certain diets can help the healing process...but that will be true only *if* a person truly wants to get better and he is not sabotaging himself. My experience is that abstinence from food, i. e., fasting, has the most beneficial effect on producing healing. In my opinion, fasting is a very spiritual matter, and when done properly, there is usually a profound healing and a "spiritual gift" at the end. You have to process your mind when you fast; the mind is, after all, what makes you sick. Food is often used to suppress the very part of the mind you should be looking at. When you are not eating, you cannot go on suppressing what you need to be seeing because what you need to see will just confront you. There is a good book on fasting called *Are You Confused?* which explains all different types of fasts. You do not get hungry on the Master Cleanser, for example - and it works. There are many other books on fasting at your local health food stores.

In general, one could say that eating less is very good for you. You have much more energy to help keep you healthy. It has already been proven that you live longer if you eat lightly. It is a good idea to start cutting down and to cut down more every year. But do it gradually. Some people, however, feel a real loss if you tell them not to eat so much. They actually feel a loss of love...probably because the way their mother showed them love was to give them food. It could also remind them of the sadness of being taken off the breast. For some people, food is like a friend and they use it as a substitute for having real friends. The same is true for cigarettes. But once you get through these notions and get into another reality - the reality of eating light by choice - I think you will really like it.

Many people are just eating the same way their parents ate. They are not thinking of whether or not that is what they really want to eat. I notice that when I eat a very light meal and enjoy that, many people cannot stand it. They urge me to start eating more. They worry about me. They try really hard to get me to eat more. More of what they eat. They cannot shut up about it. They get stuck in medical belief systems that convince them that I am not going to be okay. Or maybe they don't want to face the fact that they would like to be able to eat less. (Or, at times, maybe I had them set up as my "mother".) Nevertheless, you need to experiment. Chances are, a new world will open up to you when you start thinking for yourself on this subject. Source your *own* rules!

If you are dealing with a severe health problem and

you feel that you need support from a healing diet and a strong healer, you might consider the program of my friend Michaelangelo in Milan. (I acknowledged him earlier for helping me heal gastritis after my sister's death.) He has a healing program using the highest vibration VEGAN foods along with very strong reflexology. This regime, although fanatical to some, has proven extremely effective for many. People with near-fatal diseases have been cured at his center.

You can reach him at his institute:
 Phone: 0039 02 89 50 2085 Fax: 0039 02 895 15555

CLEARING KARMA THAT CAUSES DISEASE:

In the book *Star Signs* by Linda Goodman, there is an important true story. A friend of hers was really shaken when he was told that he had contracted a rare disease, for which there was no cure. The disease, he was told, would gradually paralyze him over a year's time. What this amazing man did was to accept responsibility for his karma. He realized that in a former life, he had caused someone, or several people, to be paralyzed. The reaction of his original action was an attempt to balance the scales under karmic law, which is quite impersonal. He could have caused such a karmic debt by being a hit-and-run driver, running from the scene of an accident, leaving the victim paralyzed, etc. or by deliberately injuring someone in a sport such as boxing or whatever. He could have been one of those in Rome who threw people to the lions.

Upon facing his karmic debt, he meditated on polarity action and made a decision. He resigned from his high paying job, and offered his service for a very modest salary to a crippled children's hospital in a nearby city. He read aloud to the children, assisted them in physical therapy and even performed unpleasant janitorial tasks. He started to forget about his own illness. Three months after he took that work, he noticed that his pain was substantially less. Later, when he returned to his home town for a routine check, the doctors were amazed to find that all signs of the fatal disease had disappeared. It was a "spontaneous remission" - the medical term for a miracle.

Another example could be that of a barren woman who lifts her karma. If a woman wants a child and is told that she cannot conceive or bear a child, for whatever medical reason, there is a karmic cause for her dilemma. She may have abused children in a former life. She may have been an illegal abortionist who damaged women. So in this life, she adopts a child. A physician friend of the author told her that statistics are as high as 75% to 85% of women diagnosed as barren discover that they are pregnant *after adopting*. When a woman has learned the karmic lesson of atonement by taking in a motherless child to give it love, the karmic burden is lifted.

(Goodman, Linda. "Deja Vu." *Star Signs*. 120-121)

Perhaps you need to do some very deep thinking about this; ask yourself if you need to apply this to yourself in any way.

Once I took a young man to India to see my gurus. This young man had serious intestinal problems and, in fact, ended up with a colostomy at a very young age. He consulted my gurus about his karma. My gurus were reluctant to tell him because they did not feel he would handle the facts well. He pushed them and pushed them to tell him. Finally, one said that he had been a drug pusher in a past life and had been responsible for the destruction of the bodies of some of the people he had sold the drugs to. Later he asked me what to do. I told him to work with teens to prevent them from using drugs. He did not like this assignment and got angry, just as my teacher had said he would. In his case he was not ready to face the truth in himself. Apparently he needs more time to integrate this information.

Recently, one of my wealthier sophisticated acquaintances from the "old days" of Rebirthing was having an exceptionally difficult time recovering from her sister's death. She was getting sick herself and was suffering terrible dizzy spells (which I did not know about because I had lost track of her). Where had she gone? To an ashram! I saw her right afterward and she was healed. She said it was the best thing she had ever done in her life. Initially, I was surprised that she had gone alone, because she is very sophisticated; I did not think she would put up with ashram life. But then I remembered that she had gone to India with me years before, so she did have built into her consciousness the power of ashrams. She had taken our seminars in the old days and she had been Rebirthed. And so, her higher self remembered what was good for her. She did not complain to me once about the facilities. All she kept saying was that it was the best thing she had done for herself.

I have written much about the benefits of ceremonies and experiences in ashrams. For more information, please read *Pure Joy.* One of my great teachers, Shastriji, the High Priest, blessed me with the privilege of publishing in that book some of his speeches. In those speeches, he carefully explains how and why chanting heals you, how and why head shaving is so powerful, and why the ceremonies work.

Nobody is saying that you *have to* shave your head at an ashram. Nobody is saying that you *have to go* to an ashram, either. These are merely choices that are available if you want results more quickly. The point is: How long do you want to suffer?

Usually people do have resistance to going to an ashram. They say they don't have time, or they could not stand the conditions, etc. Well, that is understandable, BUT what are your priorities? Do you want to end up in a hospital? Once you are in an ashram, it is actually very adventurous and fun.

I don't want to give the impression that you go to ashrams only if you are sick. Nothing could be further from the truth. Ashrams are places of worship. The more you go, the better. This is also the way to stay in bliss, to stay healthy. It is also the best preventive medicine I know. People so often ask me where I get all my energy, etc. Quite often when students go with me to India and experience the ashrams where I had my training, they say, "I finally understand where you are coming from!"

Just being around the great souls who are living in

those ashrams is exhilarating. They transmit spiritual energy to you all the time. Also, Babaji has trained certain yogis to do a healing technique called JARA. You lie down and the yogi sits near you with his bundle of peacock feathers tied together. He strokes your body with those, while repeating secret mantras taught to him by the Guru. (This can be done only if the Guru says the yogi is ready and has prepared himself through a long, special process of purification.) This treatment is very effective.

There are all kinds of healing treatments available in the world. Don't limit yourself. You will find the right one when you are ready to let go. But always remember that it is very important to do the other steps first - the Truth Process and Confession.

SEEKING SPIRITUAL COUNSELING:

If you are stuck on something, it is often very good to talk to someone who is more intuitive than you are at the time. You should always trust your own intuition of course. But when you are sick, you may not trust your own intuition because you feel "out-of-it"; or you might feel that your intuition is almost shut down. That is temporary of course, but when you are sick, your ego IS roaring; when your ego is roaring, that is hardly the best time for intuition. However, you do have to use your intuition enough to know to whom you need to talk. At least you need to know someone you can fully trust who has tried that healer, that clairvoyant or that spiritual guide.

I became a great believer in trying many forms of

healing because I thought, "Why limit myself?" I have
had no guilt or qualms about consulting others when I
have been stuck...especially when it was a past life
that was affecting me and I could not see it nor process
it by myself. Sometimes I would easily figure out what
to do or I would have a revealing dream. But often I
grew impatient. Sometimes I just needed to hear what
a person who was clearer than I at the moment could
"see". One told me that I had a "karmic break" from a
past life in Atlantis where I had allowed myself to be
experimented upon with lasers for the upliftment of
humanity. Apparently we overdid those experiments.
This information helped me and I modified my healing methods accordingly.

Other times I had intense "cranial shifts" that were
not really headaches per se, but they were painful. I
knew they were important, but I had a difficult time. I
was told by a spiritual guide that I was having exceptionally intricate work done on my electromagnetic
fields, and as a leader, I had to be willing to accept the
ordeal. Had I not discussed this with a colleague, I may
have gone into a panic. I might have felt I needed to run
out and get an X-ray or something. Or worse, I might
have imagined I was getting a brain tumor like my
sister had. By having this support and feedback, I
relaxed and I learned to know my body better. I learned
to recognize the symptoms that indicated that kind of
spiritual change and how they were different from
other symptoms.

Of course, I must re-emphasize that you can get the
answers yourself if you need to. Sometimes there are
situations in which there are no spiritual guides

around. Once I did get quite scared; I thought I was getting a brain tumor like my sister had. I had terrible headaches and I became paranoid because such headaches were highly unusual for me. I prayed a lot. During the night I dreamed the following dream: My skull was cut off by someone and set aside so that I could look into my brain. I knew I was seeing my own brain, and that was rather eerie...but I needed to see it. There was absolutely no tumor there, but there was a place where there was "drainage" and a piece of gauze was over that. In my dream I shouted, "What is THAT?" The answer came as this: "That is the negative thought you have had that 'something is wrong with you'.... That negative thought is draining out." I was pretty calm during the dream, but later I found it shocking that I had seen my own brain. Then I became grateful. I knew that was a gift.

THE ASHRAM AS A PLACE TO BE HEALED:

Since you are reading this book, I assume you are committed to self-healing; and you are willing to do anything to stay out of hospitals, if possible! Let's hope you never create anything really serious; on the other hand this can happen to the best of us, especially during very stressful times.

If you really want to expedite the process of healing - especially if you think it is not working or is going too slowly - I would suggest you get yourself to an ashram. If you are not up to going to India, there are also many in the West.

You can also call this number for information:
719-256-4108

An ashram is a place set aside especially for purification. It is usually in a location that is rather remote
and "out in the elements" where you can receive more
spiritual power. The central focus is a temple in which
you pray, meditate and chant many hours a day. The
important thing about an ashram is this: Not only do
you have the energy available, thanks to the Guru's
grace and location, you also have a totally different
routine which is so different that it makes your ego
collapse. Often this is just what we need in order to
break up the pattern of sickness. Staying home, going
through the same old routine day-in and day-out, is
often too "soft" and in many cases will not move the
ego out. But when you are forced to participate in a
routine that is totally different, in a setting that is totally
different, you change...you are released...especially if
the spiritual energy is strong enough. The rituals and
ceremonies at an ashram help cleanse and purify your
mind and body.

The subtle ego is very hard to conquer, especially by
only your own effort. A Guru can transform your mind
into a powerhouse of inexhaustible energy. You feel
safe enough and strong enough to win the battle of
your ego in an ashram. For example, I have seen people
who were stuck in a lot of anger, which was destroying
their bodies. But they were afraid to give up the anger
because they had it wired up that they "needed" anger to
survive. (So, they thought they would die if they gave
up their anger.) Of course, this is irrational, and the

opposite is true, but the ego had them tricked. In daily life they had been too scared to drop their anger. And yet, at an ashram they felt so safe that they became like lambs... sweetest things imaginable. There, for the first time in their lives, they felt safe to give up anger.

I have seen people heal themselves of major life-threatening illnesses in an ashram. The constant spiritual energy pushed them through it. I have said the following repeatedly, and I still stick with this statement: If I had a serious illness, I would immediately go to an ashram and shave my head. I have done this even for illnesses that some people would not call serious...but for me they were conditions that were hard to heal. So, rather than struggling and struggling with my ego, I merely shaved my head. This definitely brought everything to a "head"!

Interesting Things I Have Read About Healing

"Sickness always has an element of escapism in it."
(Dr. Deepak Chopra. *Unconditional Life*. p.9)

"Complete healing depends on the ability to stop struggling."
(Dr. Deepak Chopra. *Unconditional Life*. p.24)

"Spiritual connection is the hidden variable in health."
(Ferguson, Marilyn. "The Paradigm of Proven Potentials." *New Sense Bulletin*.)

"In almost all such cases involving cancer, spiritual and psychic growth is being denied or the individual feels that he or she can no longer grow properly in personal, psychic terms. This situation then activates body mechanisms that result in the over growth of certain cells. The individual forces an artificial situation in which growth itself becomes physically disastrous. This is because a blockage has occurred. The individual wants to grow in terms of personhood, but is afraid of doing so. Often the person feels like a martyr (to his or her sex, for example) and is "unable to escape".
(Roberts, Jane. *The Nature of the Psyche: Its Human Expression*. A Seth Book. p.71)

"In cancer, a normal working cell decides that it no longer wants to function in contribution to the whole. Instead of being part of the support system, the cell

goes off and builds its own kingdom. That's a malig-
nancy."
(*Return to Love* by Marianne Williamson)

The point being made is that this is merely a reflection
of our making an ego, a separate self, a false self to
replace God.

Two examples of great information from the great
book *NEW CELLS, NEW BODIES, NEW LIFE* by
Virginia Essene:

"In brief, you are in a Holy Coordinate Point. Let me
assure you that these incoming energies bring healing
to your soul and physical genetic body patterns. For
this healing to happen, the cells must receive and retain
more Light and be released of many past restrictions,
limitations, and imperfections caused by the present
life. The paired chromosomes must be cleansed at least
four generations back." (P. 2-3 from chapter by Christ
Jesus)

"Health is an area in which everyone needs to claim
responsibility for themselves. You DO have power over
your body. From infancy you were told that you have
no power over your body. You were told that you must
always check with someone else about health and well-
being. You have the innate ability to take charge of your
body. You DO replicate your body daily. You create the
same body because you expect to see the same body. If
you wish to change it, simply intend that when you
wake up there is something new to greet you." (p. 178)

Rejuvenation - Mental Level:
  On the mental level, bringing forth immortality means releasing all the ingrained limiting beliefs about your body and replacing them with unlimited truth.

Affirmation:
"I now give up death. I give up all aging of the body, all illness and any other effect that limited thought has had upon my physical form. I give up the idea of being any age. I am ageless and eternal. I give up funerals and funeral parlors and grave sites. I give up the idea of leaving life. I joyously accept eternal aliveness now."
(P. 68: Chapter called "Divine Self" by Joanna Cherry)

  I am hoping to inspire you to read that whole book. The last chapter has a lot to say about healing, i. e. intra-dimensional healing, sound healing, and quadrant healing. It requires personal study and is well worth it. All from *NEW CELLS, NEW BODIES, NEW LIFE* by Virginia Essene
S.E.E. Publishing Company. Santa Clara, California.

"Illness is some form of inner searching. Health is Inner Peace." (P. 15, *Course In Miracles* text)

Some quotations from Marianne Williamson's lectures and book, *Return to Love.*, which I recommend strongly:

"Disease is loveless thinking materialized."

"Health is the result of the relinquishing of all attempts to use the body lovelessly." (A healthy perception of our bodies is one in which we surrender them to the Holy Spirit and ask that they be used as an instrument through which love is expressed in the world.)

"Sickness is not a sign of God's judgment on us, but our judgment on ourselves." (If we think God created our sickness, how can we turn to Him for healing???)

"Forgiveness is the ultimate preventive medicine, as well as the greatest healer."

"Illness is a sign of separation from God. Healing is a sign we have returned to God."

"By shifting our awareness from body identification to Spirit identification, this heals the body as well as the mind."

"There is a healing force within each of us, a kind of divine physician. This force is the intelligence that drives the immune system. The Atonement releases the mind to its full creative power."

Another quote from the *"NO" LAW OF HEALING* by Catherine Ponder in the book *Dynamic Laws of Healing*:

"Denial is the first law of healing. Through denial you withdraw from your mind the negative beliefs and emotions that have played havoc with your health. If you can put a thing out of your mind, you can put it out of your body. Since denial dissolves, eliminates, erases and frees, it is your 'NO' power of healing."

Any prayer or statement that helps you say "NO...I DO NOT ACCEPT THIS APPEARANCE AS NECESSARY OR LASTING IN MY LIFE," is a denial. (In her opinion, to mentally affirm a healthy condition without first denying and destroying the negative emotions that caused your ill health, is like attempting to build a new house on a site already occupied by an old building. Say NO to an incurable diagnosis.)

Say, "I refuse to accept this diagnosis." (She suggests you do not believe anything anyone tells you about your health, unless they tell you you are going get better!) Read Chapter Two of that book for further information.

In this book Catherine talks about a friend of hers who was told that her daughter, who had speaking and hearing problems, was "intellectually disabled". When the child was four years old, her diagnosis was "developmentally delayed". Fortunately the girl was not in the room when this diagnosis was given. The mother was told the child should go to a special school. The mother told the doctor she was NOT going to acknowledge this. In fact she did not tell the father, friends nor relatives. She sent the child to a normal school and the girl did all right. At age eight the child had to have an operation. The mother was then told again that the girl would never be able to have children. The mother again did NOT accept this and told no one. Later the girl grew up as a wonderful, normal person and had two healthy, normal children.

So, the point is, you can use denial to help others!

My Summary on Healing

To you, who really want to know when you will be healed:

You will be healed when you are ready to be healed. You will be ready to be healed when you believe that you deserve it. You will believe that you deserve it when you are ready to stop punishing yourself. You will stop punishing yourself when you give up guilt. You will give up guilt when you believe that you are innocent. You will see that you are innocent when you remember who you are. You will remember who you are when you stop making up the ego. You will stop making up the ego when you want Bliss and Peace more than anything else. You will want Bliss and Peace when you are sick of being sick...and when you see what a waste of time it is to be in Hell. The choice is yours. (One teacher said you have to want liberation as much as a drowning person wants air.)

Permanent Healing is merely going back to who and what you really are. It is easy and natural; the only reason it SEEMS hard is that you have to let go of addictions - addictions to thoughts that cause the conditions. It seems hard to give up addictions, because you think that they control you and that you are not in control of them. In my opinion, an addiction is a "stubborn" refusal to give up something. It could be merely a stubborn refusal to give up a thought causing your condition. When you face your stubbornness and refusal as being something you are choosing, then you know you can choose otherwise.

The *Course In Miracles* tells you that you must say, "I see no more value in this." That means that you also must admit that you get some kind of "payoff" from your pain or illness. You receive some "neurotic value" out of this condition and now you are willing to give up that "payoff". For example, maybe you have to decide that you don't need this symptom anymore as a way of getting attention. You no longer need this symptom as a way of punishing yourself. You have enjoyed enough attention and you feel punished enough! Perhaps you have learned you can get attention in a healthier way. Or perhaps you feel you have now balanced your karma and you can go on to something else.

But what if you could forgive yourself *sooner*? Then you would not have to go to the trouble of punishing yourself for so long. To forgive yourself sooner requires a basic understanding of who you are: You are LOVE and your sins are not real. You have to know that you are not a bad person. You are actually magnificent. You are a child of God. You are Divine. You are not a sinner. Your disasters are not sins. They are mistakes. A mistake merely means "missing the mark". A mistake was a slip when you temporarily forgot who you are. God does not make your errors real...because God knows you were just having a nightmare. Nightmares are not real. The ego is a nightmare. But since the ego is not real, then the error is not real. Therefore you do not deserve to be punished and you do not need to create illnesses as a form of punishment. If God does not make your mistakes real, why should you? You do not make your child's nightmares real. Do you want your children to make their nightmares real? Of course not.

Just a review of the *CIM*:

INNOCENCE IS THE ANSWER.

SINCE I AM INNOCENT,
I DO NOT NEED TO SUFFER.

SINCE I AM INNOCENT,
I DESERVE TO BE HEALED.

SINCE I AM INNOCENT,
I CAN LET GO OF ALL THE PAIN AND DISEASE.

SINCE I AM INNOCENT,
THE HOLY SPIRIT IN ME KNOWS THE SOLUTION.

SINCE I AM INNOCENT,
IT IS SAFE, RIGHT AND HOLY TO HAVE A BODY.

SINCE I AM INNOCENT,
I CAN BE REALLY HAPPY.

SINCE I AM INNOCENT,
I CAN GIVE MYSELF LOVE AND KEEP IT.

SINCE I AM INNOCENT,
I CAN HAVE ALL THAT I NEED AND WANT.

SINCE I AM INNOCENT,
I CAN HANDLE A LOT OF ENERGY.

SINCE I AM INNOCENT,
I CAN TRUST MYSELF TO DO THE RIGHT THING.

SINCE I AM INNOCENT,
I CAN BE DEFENSELESS.

SINCE I AM INNOCENT,
I AM AT PEACE.

SINCE I AM INNOCENT,
MY BODY RESPONDS TO REALLY FEELING GOOD.

SINCE I AM INNOCENT,
I CAN NOW BE TOTALLY RELAXED.

SINCE I AM INNOCENT,
I CAN BE WISER AND WISER.

SINCE I AM INNOCENT,
I CAN SAY NO WITHOUT LOSING PEOPLE'S LOVE.

SINCE I AM INNOCENT,
I CAN ENJOY FOOD, MONEY AND SEX.

SINCE I AM INNOCENT,
I CAN ENJOY EVERYTHING.

SINCE I AM INNOCENT,
IT IS OKAY TO HAVE THINGS.

SINCE I AM INNOCENT,
I HAVE NOTHING TO WORRY ABOUT.

SINCE I AM INNOCENT,
I CAN LEAVE SITUATIONS THAT ARE NOT GOOD.

SINCE I AM INNOCENT,
FUN IS NATURAL.

SINCE I AM INNOCENT,
LOVE IS NATURAL.

SINCE I AM INNOCENT,
LIFE IS NATURAL.

SINCE I AM INNOCENT,
SUCCESS IS NATURAL.

SINCE I AM INNOCENT,
I DO NOT HAVE TO AGE AND DIE AND PUNISH MYSELF.

SINCE I AM INNOCENT,
I CAN LIVE AS LONG AS I CHOOSE.

SINCE I AM INNOCENT,
I CAN BE IN THE KINGDOM OF HEAVEN HERE AND NOW.

SINCE I AM INNOCENT,
I CAN BE CLOSE TO THE SPIRITUAL MASTERS.

SINCE I AM INNOCENT,
I CAN MAKE A BIG CONTRIBUTION TO HUMANITY.

FINAL WORD
(For now)

If you read hundreds of books on healing, the common denominator would surely be LOVE. That is obviously the secret of all successful healing.

The healer must love the patient; and the more loving the healer is, the faster the patient will be healed. But the patient must return to self-love and love for God and life. That is the key. If you are the patient OR the healer, meditate on love.

When I was working in Japan for the first time, I heard an incredible true story. I was told of a man who developed cancer of the lungs. What he did upon hearing that diagnosis was amazing. Every day he sat before his altar and expressed APPRECIATION for his lungs, for life and for God. He constantly meditated on appreciation. By doing this, he had a complete miracle healing. The healer who told me this story explained to me that APPRECIATION is one of the very highest vibrations for healing.

If APPRECIATION is the ultimate vibration for healing, imagine how it could also be preventive medicine. Perhaps if we sincerely appreciate people and things and life, then perhaps we would not even get sick. Perhaps if we appreciated and loved ourselves all the time, we would not have the problems we have.

THINK ABOUT IT!

Health in the Future

The famous trend setter and marketer, Faith Popcorn, has been called the Nostradamus of marketing. In her book *The Popcorn Report*, she talks about how we all think, work, and live in the 1990's. In this book she states that self health care is the future. We will become our own experts. We will counterpoint the advice of a Homeopathist, a Reflexologist, etc..

Faith Popcorn Predicts:
"Medical knowledge and alternatives will cross cultures in a way we have never seen before. Homeopathy, Reflexology, Acupressure and Acupuncture, Biofeedback and Holistic Medicine will move from the fringes to the mainstream of medicine. Even newer-sounding approaches such as Aromatherapy, Herbology and Ancient Indian Ayurvedic Medicine will be incorporated into traditional treatments or stand on their own as preferred courses of action." (p. 67)

Of course, it is obvious to me that Rebirthing will be included in that list! She also feels that entertainment and travel will be health and longevity obsessed.

"Beyond health spas will be "Mood Spas", Universal Energy Gyms, Mind and Spirit Reunions, including therapeutic cruises that slowly take you to healthy places, in an effort to heal your body , touch your soul, and bring you back, twice blessed." (p. 68)

She says we may not yet be ready to admit aloud that our goal is truly to live forever...but we will pay anything to stay alive. Well, I did admit out loud that I wanted to live forever when I wrote the book called *HOW TO BE CHIC AND FABULOUS AND LIVE FOREVER*. I was really daring and ahead of my time as usual. I was happy to see that she calls *"Staying Alive"* Trend No. 7. Faith Popcorn: *The Popcorn Report*. A Currency Book, published by Doubleday, September 1991.

INTERESTING TIDBITS FROM THE ENQUIRER:

Some people are embarrassed to read the *Enquirer*. Some people hide that they read it. I am not embarrassed and I don't hide it because I like to study human nature. I find paragraphs like the one called:
"Five Most Common Health Problems for Men and Women."

According to University of Michigan researcher Lois M. Verbrugge, the five most common health problems for middle-aged men are:
1. High Blood Pressure
2. Arthritis
3. Hearing Impairment
4. Chronic Sinusitis
5. Heart Disease

The five most common health problems for middle age women are:
1. Arthritis
2. High Blood Pressure
3. Chronic Sinusitis
4. Hearing Impairment
5. Hay Fever

Well, according to Louise Hay, who wrote *Heal Your Body*, the metaphysical causes of these conditions are:

High Blood Pressure:
Long standing emotional problem not resolved.

Arthritis:
Feeling unloved, criticism, resentment.

Hearing Impairment:
Not wanting to hear something.

Chronic Sinusitis:
Irritation...especially to someone very close.

Heart Disease:
Lack of Joy...hardening of the center of love.

Doesn't that therefore mean that we are a society in need in the area of love, that we are stuck in resentment and criticism and we don't want to hear?? Are we so addicted to favoring money and position that we are forgetting the most important things in life? Are we so rigid that arthritis is popular? Are we so unaware that we need to resolve emotional problems that we have to shoot up our blood pressure to get our own attention? All symptoms are for getting your attention and for waking up. The trouble with these symptoms mentioned here is that by the time you create *these*, they could be really hard to reverse. Prevention is the whole point. Wouldn't it be better to take the time to handle emotional problems before they turn into a diagnosis like these?

The whole point of Louise Hay's book *HEAL YOUR BODY*, is that you must first work to dissolve the mental cause. Her book explains the common mental causes of conditions. Carry this little book with you and pay attention. Don't become one of the statistics mentioned in the *Enquirer*. The problem with reading these statistics is that if you go into agreement with them, you can easily create them in your body. What you believe to be true, you create. So you must decide that this will not become true for you; and of course you must carry through with the Spiritual Purification procedure to prevent it.

Part V

My Most Difficult Initiations as a Healer

Going Toward the Stargate

Sometimes the challenge of being a committed Lightworker is shocking, even to me. For example, I never dreamed I would have to go through a kind of "crucifixion" in France. Actually it was a spiritual "opening" or "initiation", but it felt like a crucifixion. Oh yes, I did ask for liberation in this life - and Immortality so I should not be surprised, I guess. Also, I have an assignment in this life to be a pioneer on the "front lines", so I should not be surprised. But it would be a lie to say I was not shocked at what happened.

It was January 1st, 1992, when I started the journey. I was aware that the big day, January 11th, was coming up and I should have known I would be profoundly affected. This was networked as a special day, like Harmonic Convergence, for an evolutionary leap. Lightworkers were gathering around the globe and linking up to welcome the Dove, the symbol of Planetary Ascension. Under the direction of Archangel Michael, three stargates were to be opened, one at each pole and one satellite stargate that revolves around the equator. It could be thought of as symbolizing the Holy Trinity, as formlessness and Spirit. This I already knew from the *World Ascension Network Newsletters* and by word of mouth, through my colleagues in the Consciousness Movement. My newsletter stated that "Through the newly opened stargates flows a Christic 'super glue' that serves to hold the etheric perfect to the physical imperfect. Over the course of the decade, and in a specific order, all blueprint grids and ley lines will be set into place." Fine; I was into it. I agreed to fast on January 9th, 10th and 11th and for sure I would meditate at the agreed time, 11:11.

It so happened that around this time I had been instructed by my teacher in Spain to move to France. I was having a really hard time with this assignment because I don't speak French and I have a huge block to learning it. All my guides did agree that I needed to be in Europe during this time to help support these changes. I had always been very good about fulfilling every assignment; so therefore I set out for France to tour and see where I should locate. Fortunately, my teacher Shastriji in India had instructed one of my students, who is trilingual, to accompany me. Another student, who is French, was also with us the first half of the trip. The only directions I received on the phone from a guide was to go to Bordeaux and find a man named Peter. This mystified me. I was not given a hint where to find him. And everyone said I was nuts for going to Bordeaux. I could not tell one town from another. I knew nothing about France, it seemed. I merely told my students that we had to go there.

Half way there, we stopped to visit some people we knew. I was shocked to see them living with no central heating...only a fireplace stove. I was FREEZING. This added to my resistance which then really began building up. I felt helpless, not knowing French, and I did not know where I was going. I did get it in my head, though, that I had to find the place the Dalai Lama had visited. I had no idea where that was either, but I knew I had to go. The first night we stayed in a delightful town called Sarla. I was so cold that I had to sleep under my fur-lined coat. I could not imagine people living like this in modern times... who needs this? But we did find the Buddhist center and we did find a man named Peter there, so I felt I was on the right track. But why were my guides sending me on this route? The people I met through Peter started showing us a number of castles... They kept wanting me to see these castles from the 1200s. I thought, "Who needs this? I am a futurist." The more castles I saw, the more I went into deeper resistance. I felt forced backward in time and I hated it. By now I could not imagine living in France. I was told I needed the astral influences...but what kind of "bullshit" was that? I felt they had not given me enough information... Later I realized that had they done so, I would never have taken this trip. Things got harder and harder and harder. We would sometimes be in a little French town and be the only ones in a hotel...always freezing. It seemed that everyone ate goose liver and went to bed very early because there was definitely nothing happening.

I told Alan I had had it and I wanted to go farther south where it was warmer, and that we could stop and visit his mother. Besides, the rental car was getting too expensive and I was getting too resistant. We headed south and I was so pleased to see a glimpse of a pale sun and to meet Alan's mother that I felt happier. I could not speak a word of French to his mother, and therefore was shocked that she told him she had never been so affected by anyone's presence in her life. She did not want me to leave. I was simply amazed by her impression because I felt I was still totally resisting France. How could she feel so good about me? This kind of woke me up as to who I was again, and I felt rather guilty. Why couldn't I always be loving, no matter where I was? I had been so many places and had so much fun. What *was* my problem with France, anyway? Everything seemed too difficult. I was not used to this at all. I could not understand what was going on. I had lived in Peru in the Peace Corps and had taken Rebirthing to Russia and Ghana, Africa. So why on earth would I be this resistant to France? Finally, I could stand it no longer. I called my teacher.

I confessed it. I told him that if this was a test, I felt that I was flunking it. I told him I could not get my mind together and so on. Then he informed me that I had had a past life in the year 1213 in France and I had failed to complete my important mission because a war had broken out. I now needed to visit the area of Avignon and San Remy, where I would get a lot of "answers".

Well, I had been incredibly close to the right places. As it turned out, we had to return the car in Avignon. I had a very adverse reaction to that town. The Popes had escaped there once. I guess it is a powerful town, but for me that is where the hell really began. One afternoon, I was walking the streets as my teacher had told me to do. I was looking in a shop window and I suddenly lost my vision. Everything turned black. I was alone, and I was sure I was fainting. Suddenly I grabbed a light pole and squeezed my nipples very hard in order to stay in my body. I was swaying and I could not remember where my hotel room was. But miraculously it was right in front of me, so I ran to my room and cried hysterically. I had enough sense to realize the past life was coming up...but I had been through past lives before. Why was this one so much worse? I insisted that we get out of that town the next day. I could not stand it. I sent a fax to Spain and the whole fax arrived totally black....

We made it to San Remy in a borrowed car. The keys got locked in, so I had to stay. I could not escape this time. But I was quite interested in this town. After all, it was the home of Nostradamus. So I headed to the Nostradamus Cafe to report the key situation. It was Sunday, of course. This was complicated. There were no hotels open for the winter, of course...except an old chateau on the outskirts of town. It was very cold, of course. Alex and I checked in. Alan had stayed with his mother. So there we were...the only guests again....

That night I had a very unusual dream. It was the beginning of my opening, but I still did not understand what was going on. I dreamed that I saw a serpent, and it was cut up in pieces. Then suddenly, a painter came along and got the pieces and made it into a very breathtaking painting. The painting was so lovely that I could not get over it. It seemed to have been painted by one of the Impressionists. Well, after all, I was in that area of France.

I knew I was going to have to stay in town two days, but I was in bed the whole time. I spent the two most difficult days of my life in that chateau, which turned out to be on the property that had belonged to Nostradamus! By now it was January 7th and 8th. I was Rebirthing myself like mad, alternating dry and wet. Alex had to take care of me because my cranium had begun shifting wildly; the pain seemed absolutely intolerable. My bones were on fire to the point it was just too intense to tolerate. I could not let go of the thought, "This is too hard!" and I felt that I was going crazy. (Well, Van Gogh went crazy in that town and cut off his ear!) Alex gave me body work and I cried and cried and cried. I thought death would be easier. I told Alex that if my mind were to go too far left, I would be insane and if it went right I would die. There was a hairline down the middle that I was searching for. The ordeal began to look like the drama of Faust and the painful struggle to dethrone the ego. I had been through initiations before, I had been through cranial-shifts before and I had certainly had my bones on fire before - but *never* like this.

Then I recalled that Ram Dass said that as you get more spiritually connected, the more difficult matters come up. I had not wanted to hear that. But now that sentence was helping me to stay sane enough to begin to recite to Alex what I could remember from the *Course in Miracles*, which I had forgotten to bring with me for the first time, of course. I was able to access the lines I needed somehow. That seemed to be the only thing that kept me sane. If I had not had that and if I had had to rely on religious dogma right then, I would have been insane like Van Gogh...because that is what got him...the sacrifice and suffering aspect of religious dogma, it was said. Apparently he went mad trying to cope with that. But the *Course In Miracles* saved me instead...that and, of course, Rebirthing. Later I was told that my guides and teachers were all deliberately pushing me to the limits on purpose.

I was able to directly experience how my ego could resist a solution...the ego always does. It is like the devil tempting one to think there *is* no solution. This part of my mind made me feel utterly hopeless. But I kept on Rebirthing. That saved me. My ego began losing its supremacy, but it was forcing a huge battle. I finally remembered the part of the *CIM* that says that the Holy Spirit is the only true therapist because the Holy Spirit is conflict-free. I started shouting,

"THE HOLY SPIRIT IN ME KNOWS THE SOLUTION." AND THE SOLUTION WAS TO KEEP INVITING IN THE HOLY SPIRIT TO REPLACE MY EGO.

I remembered that the *Course* said that the ego is insane. I was having an ego attack but I did not know why until long after the whole experience.

On the third day I had had absolutely enough of that place. I told Alex we had to make it to Aux En Provance and get me to an acupuncturist. However, I could not even sit up in the car. I started sweating and my clothes became soaking wet. I was out of it. I dragged myself to this wonderful acupuncturist. When I saw him and began stripping down, I suddenly took my shirt and rang it out in front of him and the water in that one shirt made a huge puddle on the floor. I guess I made a "big splash" in his mind as well because he took it all very seriously after that. I told him I was not sick but that I was having a spiritual opening. He said he could see that. He told me that my fire energy was on total overload. He worked on me a long time.

After that I checked into the finest hotel I could find...where Cezanne used to stay. At least it was restored and warm and, best of all, one could get CNN!

Being able to see that for the first time in months helped me. I realized I was homesick. But that was nothing compared to the rest of the process. It was now January 9th. I began sweating and sweating. Alex had to change my sheets often...every hour and all during the night. I never got out of bed for two more days. By now, my teacher Jose, who was "monitoring" the whole thing, sent a message that all was well and that I had to go through this. He still did not tell me why. He said the energy I was getting would benefit me and everyone in contact with me. But I felt like killing him...literally. He was pushing me too far. It was still too much. Did he have *any* idea how much this trip was costing me? That I had nearly gone insane? That I had nearly died and had had a horrible time? I literally felt that I would *never* recover. I was stuck on that thought a whole day, too. I felt wounded, permanently injured. Alex had to take care of me every second because I could not move.

And then finally it was the 11th, the day they "unlocked the gates of Heaven". At least I had done well with fasting because I could not eat a thing for days, had I even wanted to.

At 11:11, I began meditating. The fire had calmed down. I had stopped sweating; but then I began to cry and cry and cry. I felt as though I was being ripped open, something like St. Theresa used to write about. She wrote "God has ripped me open." Frankly, it felt more like wild lions to me. I failed to see the rapture of it. I could not stop crying. That night I dreamed a man was killed by a wild lion. The father of the man was blaming the siblings for the death. I took the siblings into my room and reminded them that they were not to blame. (I was reminding myself that others were not to blame for this battle I had been through.) In the second part of the dream, I was in the Himalayas. There was white snow everywhere. Suddenly, away off up in the high peaks, I saw a huge red circle "pulsating". It was fresh red blood. I shouted, "What is *that*?" I was told it was a pack of wild lions during mating.

The day after 11:11 I decided to go to Madrid and face my teacher head-on. I was still mad at him. Alex had to go back to Barcelona. In the Marseille airport, I kept chanting, "I will not faint!" In Madrid I called Jose immediately. Surely he knew I was mad at him... because for the first time ever he invited me to his home. When I got there, he poured me a brandy to calm me down. He was so loving and humble that I completely forgot that I had wanted to kill him. Now he was saying that I actually did not have to live in France...just go there and clear my past lives. I would have sworn he had told me to *live* there. I know he did. But then, if he had just said, "Go to France in order to clear," I would have been like a tourist. I would have never gone that deep.

Then he told me he had to clear me because I had to be in charge of many healers in the late nineties when great epidemics are expected. Then he told me I was not yet "done" in France. I had to go to Portiers and I told him there was *no way* I was going back there that year. He would never tell me who I had been in that life or those lives. Maybe it was better. I felt half dead in his presence. But he kept telling me to connect with the good work I had done back then. I kept dreaming of towns in France burning during a war....

The last night in Madrid, Adolfo had a dream: He

and I were looking at a picture of Babaji. Suddenly we looked at the sun and that very picture appeared in the sun and became alive. Later we were in the house and Babaji suddenly came through the window, directly from the sun as a huge flame and entered my body in front of Adolfo. I guess I slept through that; however, Adolfo said I was filled with flames from the sun and Babaji was inside me. Then he apparently materialized next to me and began speaking broken Spanish the way Adolfo speaks broken English. (Babaji always told us that if we see him at night in a dream, he was actually there because we cannot make up dreams about an Avatar.)

The next morning Jose called to say good-bye and told me to go to where there was sun! He and Babaji were obviously in cahoots over my process! He also read a poem he had written for me...something about letting go of the "bitter taste" of that experience, obviously. So I did. But then I had to go back to France the next year.

On that trip I took two female companions with me. When we arrived at the home of Joan of Arc we became rather sick and began shaking. During that trip I was more sane and did not have to go to bed so much. However, I definitely needed to see an acupuncturist. I told him I was in town to clear my past lives. He suddenly ran upstairs and got a big fat book on the history of France and started reading to me in French about some king. I thought, what possessed him to open to that part? Was he channeling? Was I that king? Well, I cannot remember any of it except that he read to me in French one half-hour while I was under the needles. He was determined that I should know that era of French history. I did not understand what he was saying but my translator summarized it. At the time I knew it was perfect. Right now I cannot remember any of it.

After all that, I went to India. At the end of my annual trip, I was shocked to have my teacher Babaji put a tourniquet on my left arm and shout a mantra at my third eye for five straight minutes. He said he was going to unravel my mind completely. Then I went to Madrid to rest and I was flat out again for five straight days. I could not move. This time I was not going mad, but I could not move. I prayed constantly. At last help came. A healer from Mallorca walked in the door. While she worked on my body for three hours, kneading it like bread dough, she saw many past lives. Then she said I was going to have to go through the resurrection.

I was scheduled to go to San Sebastian. I could not get on the plane without help. My assistant that week was a wealthy Chinese millionaire. (I remember she was wearing Armani clothes in the Madrid Airport.) At the presentation, one hundred people were waiting for me. I could hardly stand up. I was soaking wet again. I decided I was going on stage no matter what. I started sharing in Spanish what was happening to me. Then suddenly I *was* resurrected, and right in front of them. A frightfully loud sound roared through the electrical system as if it had its own kundalini coming toward me. When that blast came out of the microphone, it had such a force that it entered my body and I jumped right in front of everyone. I was healed! I was resurrected right then and there. I still wonder what those people thought. Anyway, the Spanish people always love me, always accept me.

I spent the year recovering from that initiation. But, that year in India, Shastriji put tourniquets on both of my arms and shouted mantras again. I had this treatment three times. I should have known the next year might be even harder. *HARDER?* What an understatement! My final initiation was the hardest thing in my whole life.

Initiation into the Void

It was December 1, 1994, eleven days before the important evolutionary leap called 12:12. On this day vibrations were altered on the earth, new amino acids were triggered in our bodies, new hydrogen matrixes, and a spiritual quickening happened, making aging and death optional. I should have known something major would happen to me. Look what had happened to me on 11:11! But I was going ahead with my plans to go to Egypt and join others who were going there for more knowledge on Physical Immortality. Since I had been there before and had taken a tour, I agreed this time to be a leader on one of the boats. Many other leaders were going, fortunately, because I did not make it.

On December 1st, I was standing before my colleague's lovely altar in Santa Fe, enjoying the essence of Quan Yin. I felt totally innocent. Suddenly a force came at me from outside my body and hit me very hard over the heart area. At the same moment, the woman of the house came down for our meeting, so I did not mention it. I thought it was unusual all right, but we continued with our meeting and I thought the effect would go away. After that meeting, I was knocked out flat at Emily's house and I could not move. But the next day I was in the car, going to the airport, anyway. I began shaking quite violently and Emily's daughter Victoria informed me she was not taking me to the airport. I said, "Oh, this is just some kundalini moving. I will be all right." But I was not all right. I could not get on the plane. I thought, "Oh, I will just go tomorrow instead."

But tomorrow was worse. I was in a thoroughly strange state. That night I received a call from a guide in Puerto Rico. She said, "A man wearing white robes has appeared with flowers for you; he is laying them at your feet and saying you are not to go to Egypt. You are to stay where you are and have your own private initiation in seclusion." Okay, I had to resign myself to the fact that I was not going to Egypt. But the main problem was not that. The main problem was that I felt like someone had grabbed my heart area and was squeezing it. The pain was almost intolerable.

I called my friend and confessed to her what had happened at her home. She said maybe I had been hit with energies from the Middle East which were flying around her house...or dark forces. I did not like that reply at all. I did not want to believe in dark forces and make them real. She said, "Well, call it the cosmic ego." That thought only frightened me. Were forces trying to stop me? I became utterly paranoid. A multitude of turbulent past lives came up in which I had been assassinated for being ahead of my time - assassinated by groups of people who had harassed me for years. They were absolutely terrifying to remember. I would lie by the fire and a heavy, overpowering energy would surround me. I became more paranoid. I felt that people were out to get me. Never in my life had I been a fearful person. I was not used to feeling fear. I could not imagine where all the fear was coming from.

All that was occurring at the same time that my whole organization was completely ripped apart. I had no support from people on my staff except for one or two dedicated members. Everyone seemed to enter into some horrendous past life that we had had together. Everything was weird, dark, torn apart. I could not tell which life I was in, who was supporting me and who was not. I felt that I could not trust anyone. I was alone and felt totally unsupported - except that Emily and Victoria, who had been at ashrams with me many times, were there for me. Diana also called me every day. Their concern kept me sane. I could not eat. I was constantly terrified...of what, I did not know.

I called Beth for help. She came over and sat with me and all she would tell me was that for two years I had been prepared for this by my teachers. It was an "Initiation into the Void". She said I had to go through it alone. Then she added that I was to open my heart to the level that Ghandi had attained and that was going to be difficult - that I had to learn to feel compassion for the whole world. I was given no more information. I felt desperate. I could not clear my body. Nothing worked. None of the old techniques were right for this process. The oppressive energy I did not understand at all. Emily would build a fire and I would lie by the fireplace and listen to the Arti. That helped somewhat. Another thing that helped was Rolfing. My Rolfer came and gave me three sessions that week. That made me feel saner. She was extremely supportive.

Sometimes I would get too much fear in my body and I would actually go and get in Emily's bed. She was very kind that way, and very stable and would just get up and be with me during the night. None of us slept much. Something had "taken over". It was impossible to figure out. I began calling some clairvoyants for help. I needed help. I felt desperate for help, actually.

People were very kind to me, but nobody could really explain what was happening. At least I was able to get help clearing the past lives coming up, especially from Janolyn in Los Angeles and Marti in Iowa. But that was only one aspect of the whole process. I cried almost continuously. If I could not have cried, I would have gone crazy. I wrote to my gurus and put the letters on the altar. One wrote me back and told me to *shake out* the fear and that was all. Obviously I was not to have much "information". I had to learn to *trust* more, and that was not easy when I felt terrible. But at least I was not sick.

Finally, on December 11th, I felt that they had had enough and I needed to give everyone in that house a break. I got on a plane and went to Los Angeles and stayed with old friends. But I was still a mess. Either I had a severe gripping feeling over my heart chakra or I had terror going up and down my spine. I had to stay very close to my friends who were Rebirthers. One day I made a decision to go to the Jose Eber salon in Beverly Hills and have a complete makeover. During this period my old friend Bobby Birdsall took care of me. At the salon he watched all the gorgeous women while I had a makeover. I figured that I was changing completely, so why not a new hairdo? These little things helped. I hung around the old timers, like Mannie and Annie who were fun. I needed *fun* - simple things to keep me in my body. During this period I could not work. I was running out of money. I had to cancel several events, including a conference in Israel. No way could I have handled Israel in that state. Being in such a condition is the worst nightmare for a performer or public figure.

But there were a few things I could not cancel. Before Christmas I had to go to Salt Lake to conduct an event in Salt Lake and attend an evening event in Portland. In Salt Lake I had a difficult time on stage, which is unusual for me. It felt as though glass was shattering in my spine. I felt that I would faint. But nobody knew and I was able to do the event anyway. When I got to Portland, I decided to sit down for the whole presentation. Fortunately, the universe agreed and provided a couch for me on the stage. I was in a church. I told the people that I had to do my devotions in public with them, because I was going through too much. That was the right decision.

During the Divine Mother prayers, I saw a lovely blond woman in the audience having a "religious experience". She was shaking and crying. I hoped that she would come and tell me about that at the break, and she did. She stood in line to speak to me; then she shared that she had seen my guru Babaji on stage with me.

"Thank God," I said, "I need to know if he said anything." She told me that he had said the following: That *I had now become the cave and he is taking off the trousers.* I understood his message at some level; but I asked her to come and sit with me at the end of the presentation, which she did. I had *wanted* to be like the cave, the womb of the Divine Mother in Herakhan where my guru had materialized his body. This meant I was becoming what I needed to become. And "taking off the trousers" meant, I assumed, that he was getting me out of the masculine side of my being to the feminine side where I belonged. For years I had had to be in the masculine side, on the "front lines" in the Patriarchal energy. Had I not, I would have been quite sick. Now it was the right time and safe enough for me to switch. This switch was one of the most difficult ordeals in my life as a public figure. I had to change at the deepest level. I had to confront every one of my fears of being a female leader. Being a male leader was easier. I had done it numerous times before.

At the end she and her mother came and sat with me. The Mother had the same name as I: SONDRA. How symbolic! It was amazing. I sat across from Sondra, the mother, who just loved me, while the daughter, Oshara, a pure clairvoyant, told me the following: "There is a Being behind you who is like an alien...very tall and he is holding a long, long scroll of names of women who made an 'agreement' to allow the Patriarchy to take over." "Obviously to balance the karma of the Matriarchy", I thought.

She said that he was telling me that I had to be the one to break this pact. I had to decide if I was willing to take this responsibility. Then he disappeared and she told me I would have to face him later. I took this as another test to see if I was, after all I had endured, still willing to take the responsibility for the Divine Mother Movement.

I returned to Los Angeles. In the home of Dana and Peter I was confronted with "the being" again. He appeared to me one night. He was tall and his ears were different from human ears. I stood up to him and agreed. I woke up in a cold sweat. I was terrified again. These experiences were over my head. I had to call Ashanna for help. She kept telling me that I was stronger than my fear, which was the right thing to say.

I decided I needed a vacation for the New Year. I went to Puerto Rico because 1) it was warm and 2) my friends there were getting married. I got a house on the beach...but the process continued. There was no escape. I had thought that I would be able to hide in Puerto Rico. What a joke! I went to the wedding on New Year's Eve Day. However, at the door I was greeted with the news that the groom's brother had died three days before. Since people were arriving (Can you imagine?), we carried on. Half the family knew and half did not. I was not to tell the mother. I sat in the kitchen and half the family that knew would come in and tell me they had terrible headaches, etc. It was a trying time for everyone. The next day at the "celebration" the caterers arrived with everything. Half the family felt they should cancel the party. The other half said to go ahead. I was sitting by the pool. The tension was intense. *I* wanted to celebrate the wedding.

Then a man from the States came in to this party. He was in love with a Puerto Rican woman who had just broken up with him. I knew none of that. He was intoxicated, having drunk several bottles of champagne before arriving. He called me over to sit with him and then attacked me directly in a very severe way, verbally. I reminded myself not to process a drunk, and I got up and left for the back bedroom. But it did make me cry since he called me a real bitch for "changing everything", which was affecting his friend apparently. Then five other women he had attacked also came in crying! I told the woman who had been with him not to go home with him because he would probably be very violent. I felt very protective of her and I arranged for her to stay elsewhere. That turned out to be a good move because he did then destroy her apartment. It was very important to us both that I could protect this student of mine; however, I felt that I was still manifesting some past-life energy by creating the attack.

So this was a doomed wedding, so to speak. I went back into seclusion. I decided I should not go out. Emily flew down to stay with me. I had another round of paranoia in Puerto Rico. It was an expensive vacation to be feeling paranoid. One thing that helped was that Kate, a Rebirther there, took us deep into the rain forest and we did cold water Rebirthing in the natural spring pools. After my cold water session, I went into the woods and started screaming. I was getting angry at this "process" from which there was no escape.

At the airport, I was so disorientated with fear that I lost my plane ticket and almost did not get out of Puerto Rico. People were returning from New York City to Puerto Rico and everything was a mess at the airport. My bags were checked to New York City and not all the way to Los Angeles...another mistake because of my having to replace my ticket. I stood in the New York City airport with all the Puerto Ricans, having to wait for my luggage which was all backed up because of holiday traffic. So, of course, I missed my plane. I remember the belt going around and around. There was all that luggage and suddenly there was a strange sight: A baked chicken, wrapped in foil, was going around and round. The foil was coming loose, so we all could see this chicken going around and around. We all laughed. It was so ridiculous! Who was sending a baked chicken through and why wasn't it inside the luggage? It reminded me of my life right then...totally messed up, not making any sense.

I returned to California. My business partnership of 18 years was breaking apart, on top of everything else. It was no longer appropriate. Everything was changing. I saw that I was being forced to let go of everything. My old persona was dying. Was I daily, then, attending my own funeral? Nothing made any sense. I was so happy that I had read Muktananda's book *Play of Consciousness*. I remembered what he had gone through in his "training". He would, at times, just fall over on the floor while lines of people would be waiting for him outside.

I was still waking up in total fear. But at least I learned one major thing as a healer: As long as I was willing to FEEL the fear, I did not get sick. I marveled at the fact that I did not get sick. I was going through hell, but I was well. When I stopped being willing to feel the fear, I would end up in pain. So during this period of nearly four months, I either felt pain or horrendous fear. I was in one past life after another...the ones I did not want to remember. But of course, Dr. Roger Woolger, author of *Other Lives Other Selves* had said that we must be willing to experience out the difficult past lives and experience out our shadow side.

At night I began to see new blueprints actually entering my body. It was all code to me and I did not understand it at all. In one dream I saw my own kundalini lying on the floor. I picked it up and ran through the halls of a university looking for someone to explain to me what was happening. I was told that there was a professor at the end of the hall who knew everything. There was a very long line waiting for him. When I reached him, I said, "I only need five minutes of your time." He said, "You can have ten." But then I woke up and did not get the answer from him.

This was absolutely a process for me to go through alone. I had to get my own answers...and they were not coming fast enough to satisfy me. I had to surrender and trust. It was so humbling, this experience, because I could not figure it out at all. Nor were the answers in any book. I was shocked that it went on so long. I grew discouraged. I had to continually choose to live. I remember thinking that I was having a nervous breakdown; but that did not turn out to be true at all. It was the death of my ego and it was a constant battle.

Then I had to go to Japan. I was too fragile, I thought; so I asked Diana to go with me, thank God. We were there shortly after the earthquake and one week before the gasings in the underground subways. I went a week early to acclimate. I had tremendous resistance to Japan. The little apartments made me feel as though I were in a box all the time. Then there was another major earthquake warning, the very day I was to teach Physical Immortality to the Japanese. I felt that that was my real test. Had I become strong enough to face *that* without going nuts? I told Diana we should take the bull by the horns and move right into the heart of Tokyo and start chanting. I called up two Japanese devotees of Babaji and had them over to our hotel room, also a little box. (Diana said, "We are moving from one box to another.") I felt that the earthquake actually could happen because people still had so much fear of the last one that they could have easily re-created another one. Also this one was predicted by a little boy who had super powers and he had accurately predicted the other one. I thought it might occur around three o'clock in the morning before my class. At that time, on the button, my organizers were in a taxi that was hit from behind and in front at the same time - and their heads were knocked together. They came to the class in shock. I went ahead and started teaching, not knowing if the earthquake might still come that day.

I got a different kind of earthquake. A lovely man from Canada showed up in that seminar and we had a very strong connection. (As it turned out, there actually was an earthquake, but it was under the sea.)

Fortunately for me, I was going to Maui for the next stop on my tour. When I reached Maui, glass shattered around me on three occasions that day, while all the tensions of Japan came out of my body. Maui healed me tremendously. The last night after my advanced seminar of Physical Immortality, I was lying around with the assistants. Then it did happen: A minor earthquake occurred then and there. The couch was vibrating and undulating. Actually it was quite sensual. I started feeling that I was going to make it.

And now I had to go back to work seriously. I had a long European tour ahead. But more terrifying past lives continued to come up. I had hoped I was finished... but no such luck. In Poland I had a kind of accident when I slammed the bathroom door in someone's house: A bracket came right off the door and sent me flying across the room. I landed upside-down in the bathtub with my clothes on. Then I had to return to the training session I was conducting at that time, very shaken and in pain. Fortunately, I had scheduled that past-life session in the home of four doctors. I did not need them, however, except for homeopathy for shock. That was a fairly rough training session because my co-trainer started vomiting after the birth section and my translator had diarrhea and had to run off the stage. The Polish people, however were just wonderful. I experienced the power of Poland...and never have I seen so much gratitude.

In Spain I had the miracle of being able to see Jose again. He seemed totally aware of what I was going through, as usual; and he was the first one who could adequately explain things to me. He told me that new channels had opened up in me for later work. It was very important and I had to be willing to "sacrifice for God". He told me that he, too, ended up on the floor many times and unable to work because of the changes we had to go through. I felt better after that. He helped me integrate the energy. He renewed my confidence that all was in order.

I then took a pilgrimage to the remote site of the Virgin in Guarbalde, Spain, for Holy Thursday before Easter. I felt that I should fast and do penance. It was a long train ride and a long bus ride and after that, a hike uphill. I asked several people to go with me, but they could not. Again, I had to do it alone. But, after all, I had been to Medjugorje, Yugoslavia alone. I was still fragile, but I knew this would give me strength. Also, Jose had told me I would receive a "gift".

I was in a shock to find out what it is like to travel in Spain on trains during Easter. The train station was packed...like in India, body to body. I had gotten the last spot. After eight hours on the train, I changed to the bus and began a long bus ride on very curvy roads high up in the mountains. Behind me sat a woman who carried on a conversation the entire time (two and a half hours) with someone who was not there. She constantly chatted to this person next to her. I did not see anyone in that seat. Across from me was a priest from somewhere. He kept yelling at his assistant and his assistant kept yelling at him. The priest was really mouthed and terribly cranky. And yet when we stopped in a cafe for coffee, people treated him as though he were God..." Father this" and "Father that", and strangers paid for his food. He remained cranky the whole time.

When we got to the site I had thought was going to be a village, I was surprised to find that it was a mountain we had to climb. I had the wrong shoes for that and a bag that was far too heavy. I felt very critical of myself for this lack of common sense. But then I reminded myself that I had been through very stressful times, that I was fortunate not to be sick, and I could forgive myself for mistakes like this. Then I saw approaching me a little man in a pin-striped suit from the 1930's that had never been dry-cleaned, if you ask me. Well, he was terribly sweet and offered to help carry my bag. We made a funny team, him carrying one handle and me the other, since we were so different in size. I asked him if we had to climb to the top of that mountain, hoping that the site was a bit lower. He said, "Of course, madam." I finally found a *tienda* where I could leave my bag and I actually found some tennis shoes to buy in the little village we passed. Of course they did not really fit.

At the top, I stayed for quite a few hours at the site where the Virgin had materialized. I lay on the grass with everyone else in that precious energy. It was bliss, really.

When it came time for me to hike down, I had a real shock. Crowds of people were climbing up and really struggling with their breathing and fatigue, leaning on their canes or the stronger arm of another person. I saw one woman coming up carrying a huge baby. When she got closer to me, I realized she was not carrying a baby at all. She was carrying a man, only he had no arms and no legs. I wept to think of his tragic state and her loving compassion. I still cannot stop thinking of it.

Later in the chapel, during the Mass, more new energy entered my body while the priests were doing the traditional washing of the feet of twelve men. I was very glad I had come. But the problem was that I had to leave before the bus came so that I could make it back to a train that would get me back to Madrid in time. After all, a man was flying in to see me and I wanted to see him.... I decided I would hitch-hike if necessary.

As it turned out, I saw a man sitting alone in a nice car. I asked him if he was, by chance, going back to Santander. He said, "Yes," as if he were just waiting for me. Strange. He drove me to Santander in his nice car, playing nice music on the stereo all the way there. The next day the man I had been seeing for a couple years came to Madrid. I needed this break. By some mysterious "coincidence" he had just returned from Fatima in Portugal.

On this trip I also had the great privilege of meeting Mother Meera, the Indian Avatar, living in a small village in Germany. I had waited years for the opportunity and now was the right time. We had to sit three hours in absolute silence while she worked on us one by one... helping to remove obstacles. Thousands of people have come from all over the world to have her *darshan*. I had been told she was one of my main guides for the Divine Mother Movement along with Mother Mary. So I felt it was very important to go at this time. The unique gift she brings is to make available the transformative Light of Paramatman, the Supreme Being. She offers a direct transmission of this Light and obviously she is like a transformer, reducing it down in order for us to be able to tolerate it. I would recommend her book, *Answers.*

Because of these wonderful experiences with the Divine Mother, I was able to go on and handle some very tough assignments alone. Before, I had always had co-trainers, assistants or body-workers with me. This time I had to do everything alone. Even in Italy, when a blind student had an epileptic seizure during a session, I had to handle it alone; my organizers were out of the room at the time. After I got everyone centered, the assistants and students came forth to help. But basically, the tragic crisis required my strength to calm everyone. The fear in the room was very intense. I had been through so much fear already that I became remarkably calm, although I continued to have one test after another.

However, when I got to London, Diana had to Rebirth me off and on for three days. I also needed acupuncture, chiropractic and Rolfing. I was burned out. But then, when I got to the evening of my speech, I experienced such a power roaring through me that there was nothing that I had ever felt which I could compare it to. I was different. So different that I got on a plane and flew to Mallorca.

In two days I found a darling chalet near a lovely beach which I decided to rent for a year. I was beginning my new life.

APPENDIX

Healing Stories

There are so many case histories of miracles in Rebirthing that those alone could fill a book. I have chosen two reported by a nurse who is a Rebirther, not only because I am an ex-nurse myself, but because this report makes a bridge with medicine. These two Rebirthings are written by Nancy Coulter Albertson, who is an excellent nurse and Rebirther.

Case I:

My very first paying client as a Rebirther was a patient in a Cardiology Research Clinic where I was a nurse. She was also a nurse who had Stage III congestive heart failure as determined by chest X-ray, echocardiogram and physical examination. She came to our clinic to receive an experimental drug touted as the new "wonder drug" for congestive heart failure, and the only way she could receive it was to be in the research study to determine the drug's effectiveness. She saw Sondra Ray's book, *Loving Relationships*, on my desk and asked if she could read it. When she returned it, she asked if I could Rebirth her. I asked the doctor conducting the study if this would interfere in the study results. He said, "It won't make any difference" and gave me permission.

I Rebirthed her ten times - once a week for ten weeks. Every other week she received an exercise tolerance test, blood work, and an echocardiogram at the clinic. On her seventh Rebirthing, her Rebirth began with her chest tight and some difficulty breathing. As she continued, she began experiencing more and more anger. As the energy in the Rebirth reached its peak, she said she was enraged at the doctor she felt had killed her Mom. (Her mother had worked devotedly for a cardiologist... long hours, no lunches, etc. and died in his office of heart attack...alone, after hours.)

I said, "Can you forgive him for that?"

When she finally said, "Yes," her breathing relaxed, and she had a release of energy...a relaxation response... her muscles relaxed, a slight sweat spread over her body, her face looked at peace...and she felt a slight tingling all over. She continued to breathe for another 45 minutes. Subjectively, when she completed, she said she felt better than she had in years.

The next week she came to the clinic for her regular echocardiogram, blood work and exercise tolerance test. All had improved greatly. The cardiologists were so impressed with the improvements in her echocardiogram, they called the director of the study, and the company that was funding the study to report this quantum improvement. At the time, my client was on the double-blind phase of the study. This means she was either on the placebo (fake) or the drug. We did not know which she was on. The company did not know either. The codes were sealed; only in an emergency or by permission of the company could the seal be broken.

The company and the cardiologists decided the

code should be broken because if she was on the drug (and they thought she was) this would be an indication that the drug worked...and an encouraging sign which could be reported to the FDA. When the code was broken, we found that she had been on the placebo. All the cardiologists were confused and disappointed. She and I were elated because this meant that the letting go of the grudge in her heart had created a permanent healing.

Case 2:

Mrs. S. was referred to me for Rebirthing by an acupuncturist. She had been to doctors for years for a headache she could not get rid of. The only time she was not conscious of the headache was when she was under general anesthesia or asleep, and she could not sleep much because of the headache.

When Mrs. S. and her husband arrived, he wanted to come into the session. I permitted him to do so. Upon questioning, she explained that she had experienced a continuous headache for thirty five years! She remembered that it had started when they were hiding from the Germans in Nazi Germany...and she was cooking over a very smoky open stove with no ventilation in the room. At first she thought that the smoke had started the headache. Her history revealed she had been like a princess before the Nazi occupation...very wealthy, palatial homes, servants, beautiful clothing, and expensive possessions. While she was cooking, she secretly blamed her husband for her losses and when the headache started, she had been "bitching" at him.

As the Rebirth started, she wanted to keep her eyes open at first, then she gradually closed her eyes, connected her breathing and relaxed. Tension would build up in her face, so her face was almost a grimace. Then I would say, "You can forgive yourself for that." Then she would relax...her features would become calm and she would continue to breathe easily. This cycle was repeated seven to ten times in the two hours she was being treated. At the end of the session, she was tingling slightly and had no headache. She was afraid to move at first because she did not want to start it again. Eventually, she did move, sat up, walked around. She went to the bathroom and came out singing in German. She danced around the house. The headache was gone and stayed gone.

Note: Every Rebirther could write stories like these. Perhaps we should have kept records of everything. Sometimes I regret not doing that. However, it became ordinary after a while for us to see these miracles. (The *Course In Miracles* does say, "Miracles are ordinary. When they do not occur, something has gone wrong.")

For me, the dramatic healings I have seen are too numerous to mention. And I am only one Rebirther in the world. I once treated a woman who had had facial paralysis for thirteen years. The paralysis was healed before my eyes in her first Rebirthing. I saw a man who could not hear restore his hearing after he forgave his obstetrician for damaging his ears with forceps when he was born. There was one woman whose eyes were crossed *at birth* and she uncrossed them.

Rebirthers have many stories like this to tell. Rebirthers are, in general, humble people who are paid very little. They do not desire to brag about their accomplishments, simply because they do not want to sound like they take "credit" for them. Rebirthers know that these miracles have to do with Divine Energy and the ability of the client to let go into that energy.

A Tribute to Network Chiropractic
(*Spinal Analysis)*

Since Network Chiropractic, and its more recent evolution into Network Spinal Analysis (N.S.A.) is fairly
new on the planet, I unfortunately did not have access
to it when I was having to heal myself of the disease
processes which are mentioned in the book. I am sure
that I could have avoided some of those illnesses by
having had this work sooner, and I am sure I would
have healed myself much faster had it been available
then. To you readers, I say this: You are very fortunate
that this is available NOW for you.

The way that I found out about Network Care is
interesting in itself. I was staying on Maui, Hawaii with
another healer named Ashanna. We were discussing
how we could help more people quickly to be healed,
including ourselves. The question for God was this:
"How can we release the addiction to the past in the
cells more quickly, in addition to Rebirthing?" I told her
that this question was so advanced and so important
that I would have to meditate in the fetal position and
ask my guru Babaji. I was pleading for the answer and I
was finally demanding it. The answer I got was this: "It
is all in the spinal fluid." I had no idea of what to do
with that answer, but, by a miracle, the next day I got to
see how it works.

I had my first experience with Network in a group!

A local chiropractor arrived at the house with eight
adjusting tables. This was exciting to me as it had elements
similar to a group rebirthing. Chiropractors utilizing

Network are definitely in the new paradigm and are doing, in my opinion, advanced evolutionary work. They help the body release tension in the spinal cord and the meninges (the wrapping of the spinal cord which is reported to carry the tone of past stress). Through these meninges flows the spinal fluid which nourishes the brain, spinal cord and nerves. As the tension at the spine is released, it removes interference to the nerves and frees the spine increasing the flow of fluid and energy.

I felt an instant release and I could breathe and integrate the change while he moved to work on another person before returning to my adjusting table for the next gentle adjustment (touch). Later I began to understand why this kind of "clear out" adjustment is so powerful. One is directly freeing the life force itself. To me this was very dynamic as it went hand in hand with rebirthing. Yogis acknowledge the breath and the spine as major channels for the expression of the life force. I could start the breathing on the table and, afterward, it was very easy and great to get Rebirthed. I began to experiment with the idea of having these new chiropractors work during my Physical Immortality Intensive. There I decided to offer NSA every year to help people release the death urge when I teach the course in Maui in March.

During the following two years, I began to search out Network practitioners wherever I travelled. I found that the work has a strong "cumulative" effect. Like Rebirthing, the more you do it, the deeper and better it gets. Besides, people under continuous care frequently told me that they appeared to stop aging , were losing weight easily and having many miracles. I felt ready to write the founder, Donald Epstein, and tell him what a fan I was of the work and that I felt it was my duty and privilege to communicate to the world the blessings of this work. My colleague, Sharda, and I went to his home in Boulder, Colorado and also met his wife Jackie. They experiencedRebirthing and we discussed the possibilities of how we could all serve each other and work together. I have also begun rebirthing the chiropractors with whom I have become friends.

This work is now being professionally studied at the medical college of the University of California in Irvine where very sophisticated research is being done. The researchers have already documented increased flexibility, reduced stress, increased feelings of well being, an improved quality of life and the ability to listen to the inner voice.

If you would like information, contact the Association for Network Chiropractic for the name of a doctor that is doing this new work.

Association for Network Chiropractic
444 North Main Street
Longmont, Colorado 80501
phone: 303 678-8101
   fax: 303 678- 8089

In addition to acknowledging the founder, Dr. Donald Epstein, I would personally like to thank the following chiropractors who have especially given me exquisite care:

Dr. Donald Epstein - Founder (Boulder, CO)
Dr. Michael Stern (Long Beach, CA)
Sharon Stern   (Minneapolis, MN)
Dr. Hari Hari Khalsa (Los Angeles, CA)
Dr. Judy Scher (Santa Fe, NM)
Dr. Seth Friedman (Santa Fe, NM)
Dr. Emily Zapernick (Dallas, TX)
Dr. Robert Edelhauser (Virginia)
Dr. Russ Rosen (Hawaii)
Dr. Kate Kirby (Santa Monica, CA)
Dr. Sivana Hill (Laguna Beach, CA)
Dr. Jose Santiago (Puerto Rico)

For questions about Sondra Ray or Rebirthing in your area, call: 1-888-285-6762

For information on the Loving Relationships Training, call: 505-896-0413

For information on the India Quest, call: 402-697-0330

For information about Sondra Ray's many other books, contact:

Celestial Arts
P.O. Box 7123
Berkeley, CA 94707

or:

Medicine Bear Publishing
P.O. Box 1075
Blue Hill, ME 04614